Parkinson's Disease - Advances in Treatment

Edited by Liam Chen

Published in London, United Kingdom

Parkinson's Disease - Advances in Treatment
http://dx.doi.org/10.5772/intechopen.1011195
Edited by Liam Chen

Contributors
Abdullah Andaç, Akın Akakın, Emre Ünal, Ivy Zhou, Jarosław Cholewa, Jie Zhou, Joanna Cholewa, Liam Chen, Nicholas Sookhoo, Valeska Kouzak

First published in London, United Kingdom, 2026 by IntechOpen
IntechOpen is the global imprint of INTECHOPEN LIMITED, registered in England and Wales, registration number: 11086078, 167-169 Great Portland Street, London, W1W 5PF, United Kingdom

For EU product safety concerns: IN TECH d.o.o., Prolaz Marije Krucifikse Kozulić 3, 51000 Rijeka, Croatia, info@intechopen.com or visit our website at intechopen.com.

British Library Cataloguing-in-Publication Data
A catalogue record for this book is available from the British Library

Parkinson's Disease - Advances in Treatment
Edited by Liam Chen
p. cm.

This title is part of the Nervous System and Mental Health Book Series, Volume 7
Series Editor: Toshikazu Shinba

Print ISBN 978-1-80631-934-3
Online ISBN 978-1-80631-933-6
eBook (PDF) ISBN 978-1-80631-935-0
ISSN 3050-2985

If disposing of this product, please recycle the paper responsibly.

IntechOpen Book Series

Nervous System and Mental Health

Volume 7

Aims and Scope of the Series

Mental health is frequently linked to the nervous system. Conversely, disturbances in the nervous system often lead to mental health problems. However, this linkage is not as clear as it is commonly accepted. Mental health is usually described using subjective terms, which are based on psychological and psychiatric symptomatology. Diagnosis of a mental illness is made through the presence of the subjective symptoms characterizing the illness.
On the other hand, the nervous system has been deeply investigated using objective measures, including molecular, genetic, imaging, pharmacological and physiological ones. It is essential to combine objective views of the nervous system with subjective perspectives on mental health to develop an integrative approach to understanding human cognitive functions and achieving overall well-being. In this book series, experts in various fields of the nervous system and mental health will present their views on these challenging topics.

Meet the Series Editor

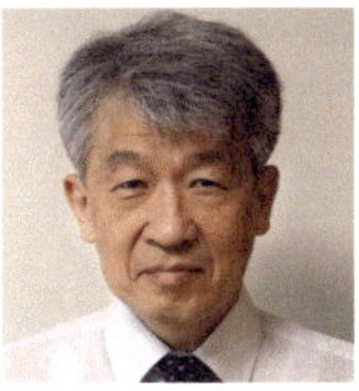

Dr. Toshikazu Shinba is a psychiatrist and neuroscientist who has been working in both clinical and basic research fields. He has been affiliated with the Tokyo Institute of Psychiatry, Department of Neurophysiology and Stress Disorders Project, and now works as a psychiatrist at Shizuoka Saiseikai General Hospital, Department of Psychiatry. The primary focus of his research is the electrophysiological analysis of attention and arousal in both humans and rodents. In clinical research, EEG, heart rate variability and skin conductance have been measured in mental disorders and arousal/consciousness disturbances. In basic research, single neuronal firing and EEG recordings have been assessed in rats. His research interests cover physiological rhythms related to attention, arousal, and consciousness in both the central and peripheral nervous systems, with a focus on understanding mental states.

Meet the Volume Editor

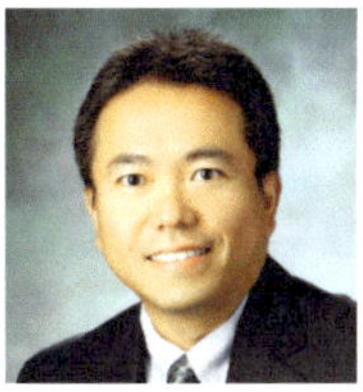

Dr. Liam Chen is a Professor at the University of Minnesota Medical School and Director of the Neuropathology Division and Neuropathology Fellowship Program. He is board-certified in anatomic pathology, neuropathology, and molecular genetic pathology. His clinical and research work focuses on neuropathology, molecular diagnostics, neurodegenerative disease, and central nervous system tumors. He has authored more than 100 peer-reviewed publications, served in major editorial roles, and contributed to multiple edited books. His achievements include national and international awards for research, teaching, and translational work in neurodegeneration and neuropathology.

Contents

Preface

Parkinson's disease is commonly associated with tremor, stiffness, slowed movement, and balance changes. However, for patients, families, caregivers, and healthcare professionals, the condition is often much broader than its most visible motor symptoms. It can affect mobility, cognition, mood, and overall quality of life. Because of this complexity, Parkinson's disease requires more than one form of care. Medication, physical activity, psychological support, and advanced therapeutic technologies may all play important roles at different stages of the disease.

This edited volume brings together a focused collection of chapters that reflect this broad and evolving approach to Parkinson's disease. The chapters in this volume present Parkinson's disease as a condition that requires comprehensive, flexible, and multidisciplinary care. The volume begins with physical function and rehabilitation, then moves to cognitive and emotional symptoms, followed by deep brain stimulation as a major therapeutic approach, and finally to advanced stimulation strategies for complex motor presentations. This sequence reflects the wide range of challenges faced by people with Parkinson's disease and the wide range of tools now being explored to address them.

Written for readers from diverse backgrounds, including students, clinicians, researchers, caregivers, and interested members of the public, this volume is not intended to present a single solution but to provide readers with a clearer understanding of the many approaches now shaping the field. We hope this volume encourages continued curiosity, collaboration, and compassion in the study and care of people affected by Parkinson's disease.

Liam L. Chen
Department of Laboratory Medicine and Pathology,
University of Minnesota School of Medicine,
Minneapolis, USA

Chapter 1

Introductory Chapter: Recent Advances in Parkinson's Disease

Liam Chen

1. Introduction

Parkinson's disease (PD) is no longer understood solely as a movement disorder. Although bradykinesia, resting tremor, rigidity, and postural instability remain central to the clinical picture, they represent only one part of a broader neurodegenerative process. Recent research describes PD as a progressive, multisystem, and biologically diverse condition. Nigrostriatal dopamine loss remains a defining feature of symptomatic disease, but it occurs alongside alpha-synuclein misfolding, mitochondrial stress, lysosomal and autophagy impairment, neuroinflammatory signaling, inherited susceptibility, and environmental influences [1–3]. This expanded model has shifted the field away from a narrow focus on treating motor symptoms after diagnosis and toward earlier detection, biological stratification, and therapies aimed at the mechanisms that drive disease progression.

2. Current view of PD

One of the most important changes in the field is the growing emphasis on prodromal and nonmotor manifestations. Many patients develop constipation, hyposmia, mood symptoms, rapid eye movement (REM) sleep behavior disorder, autonomic dysfunction, pain, or subtle cognitive changes years before classic parkinsonism becomes obvious [1, 3]. These symptoms are not simply secondary complications; they suggest that PD may involve the gastrointestinal tract, olfactory pathways, autonomic and enteric nervous systems, immune responses, and cortical networks before the motor syndrome is fully established. The gut–brain hypothesis builds on this observation by proposing that, in at least some patients, abnormal alpha-synuclein may emerge in peripheral tissues and then spread through connected neural pathways. At the same time, PD is unlikely to follow a single biological route in every patient, which helps explain why clinical trajectories vary so widely.

Genetic discoveries have strengthened this more heterogeneous view. Variants in SNCA, LRRK2, GBA1, PRKN, PINK1, and DJ-1 connect PD with pathways such as alpha-synuclein processing, lysosomal function, mitochondrial quality control, and immune regulation [2, 3]. These genes do not reduce PD to a purely inherited disorder, but they reveal mechanisms that can shape risk, age of onset, symptom pattern, and potential therapeutic response. As a result, PD is increasingly viewed as a spectrum of related disorders shaped by aging, genetic background, environmental exposure, and biological subtype, rather than as one uniform disease.

3. Advances in diagnosis and therapy

Diagnosis remains primarily clinical in everyday practice. Clinicians still identify PD by the presence of Parkinsonism, especially bradykinesia with either tremor or rigidity, while excluding drug-induced, vascular, atypical, and other causes of similar symptoms [1]. A clear and sustained response to levodopa remains an important supportive feature. The limitation of this approach is timing: By the time motor signs are clinically apparent, substantial neuronal injury has usually already occurred. This has made early and biologically grounded diagnosis a major research priority.

Biomarker development is, therefore, reshaping how PD is defined for research and, eventually, for clinical care. The neuronal alpha-synuclein disease framework organizes disease around measurable alpha-synuclein pathology, dopaminergic dysfunction, and biological staging rather than clinical observation alone [4]. Alpha-synuclein seed amplification assays are especially promising because they can detect misfolded alpha-synuclein in cerebrospinal fluid or tissue samples. Other tools, including dopaminergic imaging, selected genetic testing, skin biopsy, blood-based markers, and digital measures of gait, speech, handwriting, sleep, or wearable movement patterns, may help identify disease earlier and track progression more precisely [5]. For now, these approaches should be understood as complements to careful clinical judgment rather than replacements for it, because they still require standardization, validation, and interpretation across diverse patient populations.

Treatment has also advanced, even though most established therapies remain symptomatic. Levodopa continues to provide the strongest improvement for motor symptoms and remains the foundation of PD treatment [1, 2]. Dopamine agonists, monoamine oxidase-B (MAO-B) inhibitors, catechol-O-methyltransferase (COMT) inhibitors, amantadine, and carefully selected anticholinergic therapy may be added depending on age, symptom burden, functional goals, and adverse-effect risk. Deep brain stimulation of the subthalamic nucleus or globus pallidus internus can substantially reduce motor fluctuations and dyskinesia in appropriately selected patients, but it does not halt the underlying neurodegenerative process [1, 2]. Long-term treatment can also create new clinical challenges, including wearing-off, hallucinations, impulse-control disorders, and levodopa-induced dyskinesia. Research on neuroplasticity helps explain this complexity: Compensatory circuit changes may initially preserve motor function, while later maladaptive changes in corticostriatal networks may contribute to abnormal movement patterns [6].

Nonpharmacological care is now considered a central part of PD management rather than an optional supplement. A large Cochrane review found that multiple forms of physical exercise can improve motor severity and quality of life, without showing that one single exercise type is best for all patients [7]. Exercise may also support balance, sleep, mood, cognition, cardiovascular health, and independence. Because nonmotor symptoms often determine quality of life as much as tremor or rigidity, comprehensive care also includes speech therapy, occupational therapy, fall-risk reduction, nutrition support, constipation management, sleep care, and mental health treatment. This broader treatment model reflects the current understanding of PD as a whole-person disease that requires multidisciplinary and individualized care.

The future goal is disease modification. Gene therapy studies are testing strategies that deliver dopamine-synthesis enzymes, modulate GABA-related targets, provide neurotrophic support, address lysosomal genes such as GBA1, or reduce alpha-synuclein expression [8]. Stem cell approaches seek to replace lost dopaminergic neurons and rebuild dopamine signaling in the striatum, with induced pluripotent stem cell technology creating new possibilities for patient-specific or standardized cell sources [9]. These approaches are promising, but they also raise major scientific and clinical challenges, including delivery methods, immune responses, tumor risks, graft survival, circuit integration, long-term safety, and proof of durable benefit.

Overall, recent advances have transformed the conceptual framework of PD. The field is moving from the late recognition of a motor syndrome toward earlier detection of a distributed biological process. Future progress will likely depend on combining clinical expertise with biomarkers, genetic and molecular subtyping, digital monitoring, and mechanism-directed interventions. The central challenge is not only to improve symptoms but also to identify the right patients earlier and match them with therapies that can slow, prevent, or repair the disease process itself.

Acknowledgements

The author acknowledges the use of GPT-5.5 (https://chatgpt.com) for language editing, vocabulary enhancement, and clarity improvements during chapter preparation. All content was reviewed, edited, and finalized by the author, who assumes full responsibility for the accuracy and integrity of the work.

Author details

Liam Chen
University of Minnesota Medical School, Minneapolis, USA

*Address all correspondence to: llchen@umn.edu

References

[1] Armstrong MJ, Okun MS. Diagnosis and Treatment of Parkinson Disease: A Review. JAMA. 2020;**323**(6):548–560. DOI: 10.1001/jama.2019.22360

[2] Bloem BR, Okun MS, Klein C. Parkinson's disease. The Lancet. 2021;**397**(10291):2284–2303. DOI: 10.1016/S0140-6736(21)00218-X

[3] Costa HN, Esteves AR, Empadinhas N, Cardoso SM. Parkinson's Disease: A Multisystem Disorder. Neuroscience Bulletin. 2023;**39**(1):113–124. DOI: 10.1007/s12264-022-00934-6

[4] Simuni T, Chahine LM, Poston K, et al. A biological definition of neuronal alpha-synuclein disease: Towards an integrated staging system for research. The Lancet Neurology. 2024;**23**(2):178–190. DOI: 10.1016/S1474-4422(23)00405-2

[5] Tolosa E, Poewe W, Noyce AJ, et al. Towards biomarker-based diagnosis of Parkinson disease. Nature Reviews Neurology. 2026;**22**(3):139–151. DOI: 10.1038/s41582-026-01185-z

[6] Popescu BO, Batzu L, Garcia Ruiz PJ, Tulba D, Moro E, Santens P. Neuroplasticity in Parkinson's disease. Journal of Neural Transmission. 2024;**131**(11):1329–1339. DOI: 10.1007/s00702-024-02813-y

[7] Ernst M, Folkerts AK, Gollan R, et al. Physical exercise for people with Parkinson's disease: A systematic review and network meta-analysis. The Cochrane Database of Systematic Reviews 2024;**4**:CD013856

[8] Szunyogh S, Carroll E, Wade-Martins R. Recent developments in gene therapy for Parkinson's disease. Molecular Therapy. 2025;**33**(5):2052–2064. DOI: 10.1016/j.ymthe.2025.03.030

[9] Mokhtari YG, Varnava I, Kyrgiannis K, Ampatsidou V, Giakoumettis D. Stem cell therapy for Parkinson's disease: A new hope for neural regeneration. World Journal of Biological Chemistry. 2025;**16**(2):106850. DOI: 10.4331/wjbc.v16.i2.106850

Chapter 2

Senior Fitness Test in Assessing the Effectiveness of Physiotherapy and Health-Focused Physical Activity in Patients with Parkinson's Disease

Jarosław Cholewa and Joanna Cholewa

Abstract

Parkinson's disease (PD) causes progressive motor impairments and reductions in functional independence, highlighting the importance of evaluating physiotherapy outcomes. This chapter will examine the use of the Senior Fitness Test (SFT) as a practical and sensitive tool for assessing the effectiveness of physiotherapy and health-related physical activity in patients with PD. It will present data showing expected correlations between SFT results and the Movement Disorder Society Unified Parkinson's Disease Rating Scale (MDS-UPDRS). Regular, health-focused exercise and physiotherapy programs are expected to enhance participants' physical abilities. The chapter will demonstrate that the SFT can serve as a convenient, multidimensional tool for tracking rehabilitation progress and improving functional outcomes in individuals with Parkinson's disease.

Keywords: Parkinson's disease, Senior Fitness Test, functional fitness, physiotherapy, rehabilitation, physical activity, MDS-UPDRS

1. Introduction

Parkinson's disease (PD) is a progressive neurodegenerative disorder with a broad clinical spectrum and notable impacts on physical functioning, social participation, and quality of life [1]. Although the disease is usually characterized by its primary motor symptoms, including bradykinesia, rigidity, tremor, and postural instability, the full functional burden of PD is best understood through what patients gradually lose the ability or confidence to do. Walking slows down and becomes less efficient; turning demands more focus; transfers require greater effort; and tasks that were once automatic begin to need conscious effort. Therefore, modern PD care cannot rely solely on pharmacotherapy and neurological examination. It must also systematically address functional capacity.

In recent years, the relationship between physical activity, exercise, and physiotherapy in PD has been clarified conceptually. Physical activity is the broadest category, including all bodily movements that increase energy expenditure. Exercise is a specific, goal-directed subset of physical activity. Physiotherapy, however, is a professional process involving assessment, clinical reasoning, personalized intervention, response monitoring, and long-term management, often using exercise as a primary therapeutic tool [2]. This distinction is important in clinical practice because the choice of outcome measures should match the purpose of the intervention. If the goal is to maintain or improve the patient's daily functional performance, then measurements should go beyond disease-specific symptom scales and include performance-based tests that reflect real-world physical abilities.

Evidence increasingly supports early and consistent rehabilitation involvement for PD, along with ongoing promotion of exercise and health-focused physical activity throughout the disease course [3, 4]. Large reviews of the literature show that several exercise types may enhance motor outcomes, gait, balance, functional capacity, and aspects of quality of life, although no single form of training can be considered universally ideal for all patients [5–7]. These findings emphasize the need for practical tools that enable repeated, safe monitoring of rehabilitation outcomes in both clinical and community settings.

The challenge in PD assessment is that disease severity and functional performance are related but not identical. A neurological rating scale might describe symptom burden, but it will not always fully capture how well a person can rise from a chair, turn, step, reach, maintain balance, or sustain effort over time. Rehabilitation, however, mainly focuses on these abilities. In that context, measures of functional fitness deserve more careful attention.

The Senior Fitness Test (SFT) may represent a useful option for this purpose. It was originally designed to evaluate functional fitness in older adults using affordable, field-based tasks that assess strength, flexibility, mobility, balance, and endurance. These same aspects are highly relevant to PD, where decline affects multiple areas and is often most evident in daily activities. This chapter suggests that, although not disease-specific and not a replacement for neurological evaluation, the SFT can offer useful functional insights into the impact of physiotherapy and health-focused physical activity in individuals with PD.

2. Parkinson's disease as a cause of functional decline

The disabling impact of PD extends far beyond a descriptive listing of its main symptoms. From a rehabilitation point of view, the key issue lies not only in the fact that a patient has bradykinesia or rigidity, but also in how these problems lead to less efficient walking, impaired transfers, poorer postural responses, reduced movement amplitude, and diminished confidence in moving. Functional decline in PD is, therefore, multidimensional and often accumulates over time. It shows up not as a single failure but as a gradual shrinking of the patient's safe and effective movement options.

Ambulatory activity is particularly crucial in this context. Long-term studies have demonstrated that a decline in walking-related activity is a key factor in disablement in PD, and tracking the course of ambulatory limitations can provide valuable insights into how disability progresses [8, 9]. Practically, patients might initially notice they walk more slowly, avoid longer distances, reduce community outings, or need more focus to navigate daily environments. These changes may happen before complete independence is lost, but they often signal a significant reduction in functional capacity.

As disease stages advance, functional mobility becomes more seriously affected. Comparative research across PD stages demonstrates greater impairment in postural control, reduced ability to sit down and stand up efficiently, higher energy costs of walking, and a general slowing of motor performance in more severe cases [10]. These findings are important because they emphasize that PD is not just a disorder of isolated motor signs but also a problem with transitions and integrated movement tasks. Being able to move from sitting to standing, start walking, turn safely, and adapt the body to changing task demands is crucial for independent living.

Balance and fall risk further demonstrate the complex nature of PD. Falls in this group result from multiple interacting factors, including freezing of gait, slower walking speed, previous falls, poor balance, and task difficulty [11]. A history of instability often causes fear of movement, activity avoidance, and secondary deconditioning, which then worsens balance and mobility. This creates a self-perpetuating cycle, where reduced activity leads to greater losses that increase fall risk.

Lower-limb weakness or decreased force production may also contribute to declining mobility and transfers. Even if the pathophysiology of PD is not mainly muscular, the functional symptoms of the disease often include difficulty rising from a chair, climbing stairs, recovering balance, and maintaining locomotion. Similarly, upper-body dysfunction may interfere with dressing, grooming, carrying objects, or managing environmental supports. Manual tasks may become slower and less coordinated, while postural stiffness and limited trunk rotation hinder effective reaching and turning.

Flexibility warrants equal focus. Axial rigidity and a limited range of movement impact posture, rotation, reaching, and the ability to adapt movement strategies during daily activities. Lower-limb flexibility affects bending, stepping mechanics, and footwear management, while shoulder and upper-body flexibility are important for self-care, dressing, and reaching behind the body. These aspects are often overlooked when PD is narrowly defined as a basal ganglia disorder, yet they play a significant role in rehabilitation.

Finally, exercising tolerance and endurance becomes increasingly important as PD progresses. Reduced endurance limits sustained walking, household activities, participation in health-promoting exercise, and the ability to remain socially active. Once endurance declines, the patient may still technically be able to perform a task but may no longer do so comfortably, repeatedly, or safely within the rhythms of daily life. This distinction is clinically significant. Functional independence is not only about whether a movement is possible once, but also whether it can be maintained under everyday living conditions.

Overall, these observations support a comprehensive view of functional decline in PD. The disease impacts gait efficiency, lower-limb strength, transfers, dynamic balance, upper-body movement, flexibility, endurance, and movement confidence.

Therefore, assessment strategies meant to track rehabilitation outcomes should capture this multidimensional nature instead of focusing on just a narrow aspect of performance.

3. Physiotherapy and health-focused physical activity in Parkinson's disease

The importance of physiotherapy and exercise in PD is now well established; however, in this chapter, the aim is not to provide a detailed classification of all therapeutic methods but to emphasize that movement-based interventions can influence the same domains that should later be monitored functionally. Contemporary management involves early, regular, and long-term integration of rehabilitation into patient care, together with linking specialist-led physiotherapy with the maintenance of everyday health-focused physical activity [3, 4].

Available systematic reviews and meta-analyses suggest that various forms of exercise, including aerobic training, resistance training, balance exercises, task-specific functional training, dance, and multimodal programs, may improve selected aspects of motor function, mobility, and quality of life in PD [5–7]. From a practical standpoint, it is especially important that the benefits of these interventions are not confined to neurological outcomes but also enhance everyday tasks such as standing up, walking, turning, maintaining balance, and sustaining effort.

Therefore, assessing rehabilitation effectiveness should not rely solely on disease-specific symptom scales. It also requires tools that demonstrate whether the patient is genuinely improving in the performance of functionally meaningful tasks. The more an intervention emphasizes everyday functional performance, the more important performance-based functional testing becomes. This is where the rationale for considering the SFT as a complementary tool to traditional clinical assessment becomes clear.

4. Conceptual basis and practical application of Senior Fitness Test

The SFT was developed as a field-based assessment to measure functional fitness in community-dwelling older adults [12]. Its conceptual foundation lies not in competitive performance but in physical independence. The test was created to evaluate physiological and movement-related abilities that support safe mobility and independence in later life. This functional focus explains why the SFT continues to be widely discussed in gerontology, exercise science, and applied rehabilitation. It is based on the idea that fitness in older age should be understood in relation to abilities relevant to everyday living.

An important later development was the creation of criterion-referenced standards designed to estimate the level of physical capacity needed to maintain independence in later life [13]. Although these standards were not developed specifically for PD, they enhance the conceptual value of the SFT by connecting performance domains to daily function. In other words, the SFT is not merely a collection of practical tasks. It is a structured battery centered around clinically meaningful domains.

The Chair Stand test assesses lower-body strength by counting how many times the participant can get up from and sit back down within a set time period. In older adults, this skill is closely linked to transfers, stairs, overall mobility, and independence in everyday tasks [12, 13]. For people with PD, this domain is particularly important because difficulty standing up from a chair is one of the most common and significant movement issues encountered during rehabilitation.

The Arm Curl test measures upper-body strength by repeatedly lifting a standardized hand weight over a designated period. Its practical importance lies in the support that upper-limb strength offers for carrying objects, self-care, and repeated arm movements in daily activities [12]. Although the test does not evaluate fine motor dexterity, it captures a vital aspect of upper-extremity reserve that can contribute to functional independence.

The Chair Sit-and-Reach test measures lower-body flexibility, especially in movements involving bending, stepping, reaching for the feet, and maintaining efficient lower-limb motion patterns. In practical terms, this domain relates to dressing, footwear management, transfers, and posture adjustment [12]. In PD, where stiffness and reduced movement range are common, lower-body flexibility may have functional consequences that exceed what a single goniometric assessment can capture.

The Back Scratch test assesses upper-body flexibility by measuring the distance between the hands when one arm reaches over the shoulder and the other up the back. Its practical importance includes dressing, personal hygiene, grooming, and reaching behind the body [12]. In PD, limited trunk and shoulder mobility can directly impact these activities.

The 8-foot Up-and-Go test is a timed task where the participant stands up, walks a short distance, turns, returns, and sits down. It measures agility, transfer ability, and dynamic balance [12]. Notably, it combines several transitional movements into a quick and practical format. This integrated approach is especially useful in situations where challenges arise during initiation, turning, or sequencing, rather than during straight-line movement alone.

The 2-Minute Step Test offers an accessible way to measure endurance when longer walking tests are not practical. It assesses aerobic endurance and the ability to maintain rhythmic movement over time [12, 13]. Endurance is vital for community walking, household tasks, and ongoing participation in health-promoting exercise.

Besides its individual components, the SFT has several practical advantages. It is low-cost, requires minimal equipment, can be performed in common clinical settings, and does not require advanced technology. These qualities are especially useful in outpatient rehabilitation, geriatric care, community health programs, and adapted physical activity environments. The battery is also sufficiently comprehensive to yield a functional profile rather than a single isolated score.

These conceptual and practical characteristics help explain why the SFT may be considered useful in PD. The domains it assesses are directly relevant to the functional limitations related to the disease, which are most often targeted in physiotherapy and exercise programs.

5. Why the Senior Fitness Test may be useful in PD

The central rationale for considering the SFT in PD is that its components correspond closely to clinically meaningful domains of functional ability, which tend to decline in this population. PD affects how a person stands up, sits down, steps, turns, reaches, maintains posture, and sustains movement. The SFT provides a structured way to observe these capacities through tasks that reflect real-life functional demands more closely than symptom scoring alone.

The Chair Stand test is particularly relevant because difficulty with sit-to-stand transfers is one of the most recognizable functional limitations in PD. A patient who has trouble standing up from a chair often experiences not only reduced lower-body strength but also impaired anticipatory postural adjustments, slower movement initiation, and decreased coordination during multisegment tasks. In this way, Chair Stand performance reflects both lower-body strength and transfer efficiency. Improvement in this test may indicate more than muscular gains alone; it may also suggest better management of a key daily activity.

The 8-foot Up-and-Go test may be even more closely aligned with typical PD challenges. It involves rising, initiating gait, turning, returning to walking, and controlled sitting. These are precisely the movement phases during which many people with PD experience hesitation, instability, freezing, or loss of confidence [11]. As a timed assessment, the test provides a practical indicator of how efficiently dynamic mobility is performed. In rehabilitation, this may be clinically useful because therapy often aims not only to maintain the ability to walk but also to improve how safely and effectively the person manages complex short mobility tasks.

The endurance component is also highly relevant. The 2-Minute Step Test offers a helpful estimate of locomotor endurance and overall exercise ability. In PD, the ability to remain physically active is often limited by fatigue, gait inefficiency, reduced confidence, and deconditioning. Since regular physical activity and structured exercise are increasingly recommended throughout disease progression [3–7, 14], a simple endurance-based test can help clinicians identify limited functional reserve and monitor whether interventions improve tolerance for sustained movement.

Flexibility components should also be regarded seriously. The Back Scratch and Chair Sit-and-Reach tests might initially seem less important than mobility tasks, but they clearly evaluate movement ranges with practical daily implications. Activities like dressing, reaching, lower-body care, turning, posture adjustments, and safe movement all rely partly on maintained flexibility. In PD, axial rigidity and reduced limb excursion may amplify the consequences of reduced flexibility. These SFT elements, therefore, expand assessment and may uncover barriers to movement quality that could otherwise be overlooked.

Upper-body function is another area in which the SFT may provide useful information. The Arm Curl test does not capture the entire range of dexterity-related impairments in PD, but it does evaluate repeated upper-limb effort relevant to carrying, lifting, and functional arm use. In a multidimensional rehabilitation program, preserved or improved upper-body performance supports independence in many activities. Functional monitoring should not overlook the upper extremities just because gait-related issues are more visually noticeable.

Another strength of the SFT is its organization as a battery. Rather than relying on a single performance marker, it provides a profile across several movement domains. This is beneficial because PD presents heterogeneously. One patient might have relatively preserved flexibility but poor agility and low endurance. Another might have acceptable endurance but significant difficulty with transfers and upper-body mobility. A multidimensional battery helps distinguish such patterns and may guide more individualized exercise planning.

The PD-specific literature on the SFT is limited but suggestive. A pilot study by Cancela and colleagues found that the SFT could be used with people who have mild to moderate PD and that the results were meaningfully related to disease severity [15]. Subsequent studies also examined associations between SFT results and quality of life, supporting the idea that functional fitness measured with this battery may reflect important clinical aspects of living with PD [16]. More recently, Cholewa and colleagues reported that SFT results were strongly associated with MDS-UPDRS outcomes and were sensitive to functional differences observed with rehabilitation participation [17]. While these studies do not establish the SFT as a definitive disease-specific standard, they provide a reasonable empirical basis for considering its clinical use.

The practical value of the SFT becomes even clearer in resource-limited settings. Not every clinic or community program has access to tools like instrumented gait analysis, force platforms, wearable monitoring devices, or comprehensive performance batteries. Clinicians still need methods to assess multidimensional change. In such settings, the SFT may serve as a practical compromise between overly simple single-task tests and highly specialized laboratory evaluations.

At the same time, its use in PD must be guided by safety considerations and clinical judgment. Patients with significant postural instability, freezing of gait, cognitive impairment, or marked fatigue may need closer supervision, rest periods, task adjustments, or omission of certain components. The battery is practical, but it is not appropriate for every clinical presentation. Its effectiveness depends not only on the test itself but also on how carefully it is administered.

6. SFT in the broader context of functional and clinical assessment

The most appropriate way to position the SFT in PD is to regard it as complementary to disease-specific scales rather than as a replacement for them. The MDS-UPDRS remains one of the most important clinical instruments in PD because it assesses nonmotor and motor experiences of daily living, motor examination, and motor complications. In the classic clinimetric study by Goetz and colleagues, involving 877 English-speaking patients from 39 centers, the MDS-UPDRS demonstrated high internal consistency, very strong agreement with the original UPDRS, and an appropriate factor structure for each part of the scale. The authors also emphasized that the most appropriate approach is to use total scores for individual parts rather than a single overall score [18]. This reminds us that PD is a multidimensional condition and that even a comprehensive neurological scale does not describe a single homogeneous construct.

From a rehabilitation perspective, however, the key issue is that the MDS-UPDRS was not designed as a functional fitness assessment. Clinical assessment determines the severity of particular symptoms and disease-related experiences, whereas performance-based tests indicate how effectively the patient performs specific movement tasks. This distinction is well illustrated by the study by Brusse and colleagues, who examined associations between the UPDRS and tests of balance, mobility, and gait in people with PD. They found that the total UPDRS score was associated with selected functional measures, including the Berg Balance Scale, Functional Reach, and Timed Up and Go, but also noted that the UPDRS alone did not fully capture functional mobility [19]. In other words, the neurological scale provides important but incomplete information about everyday motor performance.

A similar conclusion emerges from research on short timed performance tests. Haaxma and colleagues compared a Timed Motor Test Battery with the UPDRS-III in 288 patients with PD and showed that the short performance battery, which required less than 5 minutes to administer, correlated well with both the UPDRS-III and disease duration. Additionally, the test-retest reliability of the summary score of this battery was very high and, in some parts of the analysis, was not inferior to that of the UPDRS-III in parts of the analysis [20]. This study did not focus directly on the SFT, but it is methodologically important for this chapter because it demonstrates that brief quantitative performance tests can provide clinically useful information and may be sensitive to functional change.

Against this background, the SFT appears particularly relevant because it covers multiple performance domains: lower-limb strength, upper-limb strength, flexibility, agility combined with dynamic balance, and endurance. The most direct data in the PD population were provided by Cancela and colleagues. In their pilot study with 30 people with PD, participants were able to complete the battery after a minor modification to one test component, and the results indicated lower functional capacity and weaker muscular performance than in healthy peers, especially in flexibility. The authors also reported significant correlations between SFT outcomes, the UPDRS, and the PDQ-39 questionnaire, indicating that functional fitness measured by the SFT was related to both disease severity and quality of life [15].

Further evidence was provided by Urgacz and colleagues, who analyzed the usefulness of the SFT in assessing the effectiveness of physical rehabilitation in relation to quality of life. In that study, significant differences were observed between participants and nonparticipants in rehabilitation across all SFT components, with the strongest association with quality of life observed for the 2-minute walk. The authors' conclusion was cautious but clearly suggested that SFT results are related to the quality of life of people with Parkinson's disease (PD) and may assist in evaluating rehabilitation outcomes [16]. This is important because quality of life is not simply a derivative of a neurological score but results from a complex interaction among symptoms, activity, and participation.

A study by Cholewa and colleagues, published in 2021, addresses the central issue of this chapter particularly closely. The authors analyzed the use of the SFT to evaluate the impact of physical rehabilitation on functional fitness and examined the relationships between the SFT and the MDS-UPDRS in 69 individuals with idiopathic PD at Hoehn and Yahr stage II. After 6 months, they observed improved functional fitness in the rehabilitation group and strong correlations between SFT results and MDS-UPDRS assessments. They concluded that the SFT is a sensitive tool for assessing physical fitness in people with PD [17]. Although these findings require further validation across disease stages and therapeutic approaches, this study provides some of the most direct published evidence supporting the combination of SFT with clinical assessment in PD rehabilitation.

It is also useful to consider studies extending beyond those focused specifically on the SFT. In a prospective longitudinal study, Cavanaugh and colleagues found that over 1 and 2 years, people with PD experienced a decline in both the amount and intensity of ambulatory activity, while some other clinical indicators changed less clearly over time. Importantly, baseline ambulatory activity and performance measures were among the strongest predictors of subsequent daily step count [8]. Ellis and colleagues, in turn, demonstrated in a multicenter cohort study that among various domains of disability, walking-related activity limitations were the strongest indicator of worsening disability over a 2-year period [9]. These findings reinforce the view that monitoring the functional performance of tasks is not merely an additional measure but one of the most clinically valuable ways to track the progression of limitations.

Evidence on functional mobility across disease stages points in the same direction. Mollà-Casanova and colleagues showed that as PD progresses, postural control, the ability to sit down and stand up, general movement speed, and the functional cost of locomotion all worsen [10]. This confirms that functional movement tasks are clinically sensitive to disease progression and justifies the use of batteries that combine several domains of task performance within a single examination. The SFT does not cover every problem characteristic of PD, but it does include several of the domains that appear particularly important for practical functioning.

Taken together, the available evidence supports a cautious but clear conclusion. Clinical scales, such as the MDS-UPDRS, are essential for describing disease severity and its neurological features. Performance-based tests, such as the SFT, may provide an additional layer of information about how the patient performs tasks related to everyday motor demands. It is precisely this partial difference, rather than direct competition, that provides the strongest argument for including the SFT in a broader model of rehabilitation assessment for people with PD.

7. Clinical and educational implications

The clinical value of the SFT in PD is likely to be greatest in settings where repeated, function-oriented monitoring is required. For physiotherapists, the battery may help establish a functional baseline before treatment begins. A patient with seemingly mild PD may already demonstrate reduced transfer ability, impaired agility, or low endurance. Early detection of these deficits is clinically important because rehabilitation is most effective when it addresses emerging limitations rather than waiting until substantial disability develops.

The SFT may also support ongoing progress monitoring during physiotherapy and structured exercise programs. Because the tasks are relatively brief and require minimal equipment, reassessment can be performed at clinically meaningful intervals without imposing excessive burden. In PD, where therapeutic goals often include maintaining independence, slowing decline, and achieving modest but meaningful functional improvements, this form of monitoring is particularly important.

Another practical advantage lies in communication. Performance-based outcomes are often easier to explain to patients and caregivers than abstract composite clinical scores. Improvements in chair rise, dynamic mobility, or endurance are intuitively understandable and may help patients recognize the functional rationale for continuing exercise. This, in turn, may improve adherence and support shared goal-setting.

The battery may also help individualize exercise prescriptions. Poor Chair Stand performance may indicate the need for greater emphasis on lower-limb strengthening and transfer training. Reduced Up-and-Go performance may suggest a need for targeted work on dynamic balance, turning, and transition control. Limited flexibility scores may indicate the importance of incorporating range-of-motion exercises into functional tasks. Low endurance could justify graduated aerobic training and progression of community ambulation.
In this way, assessment informs intervention rather than being a separate administrative step.

Outside specialized clinics, the SFT may be useful for adapted physical activity professionals, exercise specialists, and community health educators working with people with PD in group-based or health-focused settings. In such settings, disease-specific neurological scales may be impractical or fall outside the professional scope of certain practitioners, whereas the SFT provides a structured way to observe function across multiple domains. This does not replace the need for medical collaboration, but it may support the development of more systematic health-focused programs.

From an educational perspective, the SFT may strengthen a broader understanding of what rehabilitation aims to preserve in PD. It keeps attention focused on the physical prerequisites of independent living: standing up, sitting down, moving safely, maintaining balance, reaching effectively, and tolerating activity. For multidisciplinary teams, this may promote clearer communication across neurology, physiotherapy, gerontology, exercise science, and health education.

8. Limitations and critical considerations

Any strong recommendation regarding the SFT in PD must be balanced by critical reflection. The first limitation is straightforward: the SFT is not a disease-specific instrument [12, 13]. It was developed for older adults in general and does not capture many features essential to PD management, such as tremor severity, dyskinesia, freezing episodes, medication fluctuations, nonmotor symptoms, and cognitive or neuropsychiatric impairment in a comprehensive manner. For this reason alone, it cannot replace neurological or disease-specific assessment.

A second limitation concerns interpretive variability. Performance in PD may be influenced by medication timing, fatigue, stress, sleep quality, pain, orthostatic symptoms, motivation, and day-to-day symptom fluctuations [4, 18]. If these factors are not adequately documented and reasonably standardized, comparison of repeated SFT results may be difficult. Testing under different medication states, for example, may alter mobility performance independently of rehabilitation effects.

Cognitive status is another important consideration. Although the SFT tasks are relatively simple, they still require comprehension, pacing, motor planning, and sustained attention. In patients with cognitive impairment, poorer performance may reflect a combination of physical limitations and reduced executive functioning.

Similarly, fear of falling may inhibit performance in dynamic tasks, especially if the patient is not sufficiently familiar with the testing environment.

Safety is perhaps the most immediate practical limitation. Some individuals with advanced balance impairments, frequent freezing, or substantial comorbidities may require modification of, or exclusion from, selected components. The desire to obtain a complete battery should never take precedence over safety. Guarding, task adaptation, longer rest intervals, or selective omission may be necessary for vulnerable patients.

Another issue is the still-limited body of PD-specific validation literature. The existing studies by Cancela, Urgacz, and Cholewa support the usefulness of the SFT in this population, but they do not yet provide a comprehensive validation framework across disease stages, phenotypes, and clinical settings [15–17]. Minimal clinically important differences, minimal detectable change values, PD-specific benchmarks, and longitudinal interpretive thresholds remain insufficiently established. Until stronger evidence becomes available, clinicians should use the SFT thoughtfully and in context, rather than as a definitive stand-alone marker.

There is also a conceptual limitation related to the interpretation of results. Better SFT performance generally indicates greater functional reserve, but it does not automatically imply a lower overall disease burden. A patient may improve in endurance yet remain substantially restricted by freezing of gait. Another may demonstrate acceptable strength but struggle with depression, cognitive impairment, or severe nonmotor symptoms. Functional fitness is only one aspect of the PD experience, albeit an important one.

For these reasons, the most defensible position is that the SFT should supplement rather than substitute broader multidimensional assessment. Its purpose is to provide clinically meaningful insight into functional fitness that might otherwise remain underrepresented in standard outcome measurement.

9. Future directions

Several research directions deserve priority if the SFT is to achieve a more established position in PD rehabilitation. Broader validation studies are needed across different stages of PD, age groups, phenotypes, and care settings. It remains important to determine which patient groups and clinical contexts the battery is most feasible, most informative, and most sensitive to change.

Another important area concerns responsiveness. The practical value of the SFT depends to a considerable extent on its ability to detect changes associated with physiotherapy and health-focused physical activity. Preliminary studies suggest that the SFT may be sensitive to such changes, but larger and methodologically more rigorous studies are needed to determine how responsive each component is to different types of interventions [14–17].

There is also a clear need to establish clinically meaningful change thresholds for PD populations. In routine practice, clinicians need to know whether an observed change reflects true functional improvement, measurement variability, or natural fluctuation. PD-specific thresholds for minimal detectable change and minimal clinically important difference would substantially improve interpretability.

Longitudinal studies are likewise needed to determine whether SFT trajectories can help characterize disease progression or identify patients at risk of accelerated disability progression. Given the long-term course of PD, repeated assessments of functional fitness may reveal patterns that cross-sectional assessments may fail to capture. Such research would be particularly valuable if linked to fall risk, participation measures, objectively recorded activity levels, and quality-of-life outcomes.

Comparative studies should also examine how the SFT relates to other commonly used performance measures in PD, including gait tests, balance scales, timed mobility tests, and disease-specific questionnaires. Such comparisons could clarify whether the SFT offers unique added value or whether certain components are more informative than others.

Another relevant direction concerns the possible development of a PD-adapted application model of the SFT. It is possible that not all components are equally useful across all disease stages or intervention goals. A more explicitly evidence-based approach, rather than one guided by assumptions, may improve both safety and clinical efficiency.

10. Conclusions

Parkinson's disease leads to multidimensional functional decline, affecting mobility, transfers, balance, flexibility, endurance, upper-body function, and confidence in everyday movement. Because rehabilitation and health-focused physical activity aim to attenuate or slow these limitations, outcome assessment should include practical tools that reflect functioning in everyday life rather than relying solely on disease-specific symptom scales.

The SFT appears to be a promising option in this context. Its components correspond to several domains that are highly relevant to people with PD, including lower-body strength, upper-body strength, flexibility, agility combined with dynamic balance, transfer ability, and endurance. Available evidence suggests that SFT results may be meaningfully related to clinical status, quality of life, and participation in rehabilitation [15–17]. In addition, the feasibility, low cost, and multidimensional structure of the test make it well-suited to repeated use in clinical and community settings.

At the same time, the SFT is not a disease-specific tool and should not be regarded as a stand-alone replacement for neurological assessment. Factors such as medication timing, fatigue, cognitive status, symptom fluctuations, motivation, comorbidities, and fall risk all influence how its results should be interpreted. Its primary value lies in complementing, rather than replacing, a comprehensive multidimensional evaluation.

Overall, the SFT may be regarded as a practical and clinically valuable tool for assessing selected dimensions of functional fitness in people with Parkinson's disease and for monitoring the effectiveness of physiotherapy and health-focused physical activity. Further validation, longitudinal research, and refinement of PD-specific interpretive standards will determine the extent to which this potential can be realized.

Acknowledgments

The author acknowledges the use of Grammarly and ChatGPT for language polishing of the manuscript.

Conflict of Interest

The authors declare no conflict of interest.

Author details

Jarosław Cholewa* and Joanna Cholewa
Institute of Sport Science, Academy of Physical Education in Katowice, Katowice, Poland

*Address all correspondence to: j.cholewa@awf.katowice.pl

References

[1] Bloem BR, Okun MS, Klein C. Parkinson's disease. Lancet. 2021;**397**(10291):2284–2303. DOI: 10.1016/S0140-6736(21)00218-X

[2] Bouça-Machado R, Rosário A, Caldeira D, Castro Caldas A, Guerreiro D, Venturelli M, et al. Physical activity, exercise, and physiotherapy in Parkinson's disease: Defining the concepts. Movement Disorders Clinical Practice. 2020;**7**(1): 7–15. DOI: 10.1002/mdc3.12849

[3] Ellis TD, Colón-Semenza C, DeAngelis TR, Thomas CA, Saint-Hilaire MH, Earhart GM, et al. Evidence for early and regular physical therapy and exercise in Parkinson's disease. Seminars in Neurology. 2021;**41**(2): 189–205. DOI: 10.1055/s-0041-1725133

[4] Osborne JA, Botkin R, Colón-Semenza C, DeAngelis TR, Gallardo OG, Kosakowski H, et al. Physical therapist management of Parkinson disease: A clinical practice guideline from the American physical therapy association. Physical Therapy. 2022;**102**(4):pzab302. DOI: 10.1093/ptj/pzab302

[5] Ernst M, Folkerts AK, Gollan R, Lieker E, Caro-Valenzuela J, Adams A, et al. Physical exercise for people with Parkinson's disease: A systematic review and network meta-analysis. Cochrane Database of Systematic Reviews. 2023; **1**(1):CD013856. DOI: 10.1002/14651858.CD013856.pub2

[6] Radder DLM, de Lima ALS, Domingos J, Keus SHJ, van Nimwegen M, Bloem BR, et al. Physiotherapy in Parkinson's disease: A meta-analysis of present treatment modalities. Neurorehabilitation and Neural Repair. 2020;**34**(10):871–880. DOI: 10.1177/1545968320952799

[7] Okada Y, Ohtsuka H, Kamata N, Yamamoto S, Sawada M, Nakamura J, et al. Effectiveness of long-term physiotherapy in Parkinson's disease: A systematic review and meta-analysis. Journal of Parkinson's Disease. 2021; **11**(4):1619–1630. DOI: 10.3233/JPD-212782

[8] Cavanaugh JT, Ellis TD, Earhart GM, Ford MP, Foreman KB, Dibble LE. Toward understanding ambulatory activity decline in Parkinson disease. Physical Therapy. 2015;**95**(8):1142–1150. DOI: 10.2522/ptj.20140498

[9] Ellis TD, Cavanaugh JT, Earhart GM, Ford MP, Foreman KB, Thackeray A, et al. Identifying clinical measures that most accurately reflect the progression of disability in Parkinson disease. Parkinsonism and Related Disorders. 2016;**25**:65–71

[10] Mollà-Casanova S, Pedrero-Sánchez JF, Inglés M, López-Pascual J, Muñoz-Gómez E, Aguilar-Rodríguez M, et al. Impact of Parkinson's disease on functional mobility at different stages. Frontiers in Aging Neuroscience. 2022;**14**:935841

[11] Camicioli R, Morris ME, Pieruccini-Faria F, Montero-Odasso M, Son S, Buzaglo D, et al. Prevention of falls in Parkinson's disease: Guidelines and gaps. Movement Disorders Clinical Practice. 2023;**10**(10):1459–1469. DOI: 10.1002/mdc3.13860

[12] Rikli RE, Jones CJ. Development and validation of a functional fitness

test for community-residing older adults. Journal of Aging and Physical Activity. 1999;**7**(2):129–161. DOI: 10.1123/japa.7.2.129

[13] Rikli RE, Jones CJ. Development and validation of criterion-referenced clinically relevant fitness standards for maintaining physical Independence in later years. The Gerontologist. 2013;**53**(2):255–267. DOI: 10.1093/geront/gns071

[14] Yang Y, Fu X, Zhang H, Ouyang G, Lin SC. The effect of home-based exercise on motor symptoms, quality of life and functional performance in Parkinson's disease: A systematic review and meta-analysis. BMC Geriatrics. 2023;**23**(1):873. DOI: 10.1186/s12877-023-04595-6

[15] Cancela JM, Ayán C, Gutiérrez-Santiago A, Prieto I, Varela S. The senior fitness test as a functional measure in Parkinson's disease: A pilot study. Parkinsonism and Related Disorders. 2012;**18**(2):170–173. DOI: 10.1016/j.parkreldis.2011.09.016

[16] Urgacz K, Cholewa J, Uher I, Sahin B, Cholewa J. Senior Fitness Test in assessing the effectiveness of physical rehabilitation in the context of Parkinson's disease patients' quality of life. Physical Activity Review. 2018;**6**:110–116. DOI: 10.16926/par.2018.06.15

[17] Cholewa J, Cholewa J, Nawrocka A, Gorzkowska A. Senior Fitness Test in the assessment of the physical fitness of people with Parkinson's disease. Experimental Gerontology. 2021;**151**:111421. DOI: 10.1016/j.exger.2021.111421

[18] Goetz CG, Tilley BC, Shaftman SR, Stebbins GT, Fahn S, Martinez-Martin P, et al. Movement disorder society-sponsored revision of the unified Parkinson's Disease Rating Scale (MDS-UPDRS): Scale presentation and clinimetric testing results. Movement Disorders. 2008;**23**(15):2129–2170. DOI: 10.1002/mds.22340

[19] Brusse KJ, Zimdars S, Zalewski KR, Steffen TM. Testing functional performance in people with Parkinson disease. Physical Therapy. 2005;**85**(2):134–141. DOI: 10.1093/ptj/85.2.134

[20] Haaxma CA, Bloem BR, Borm GF, Horstink MWI. Comparison of a timed motor test battery to the Unified Parkinson's Disease Rating Scale-III in Parkinson's disease. Movement Disorders. 2008;**23**(12):1707–1717. DOI: 10.1002/mds.22197

Chapter 3

Neurofeedback for Non-Motor Symptoms in Early Parkinson's Disease: Cognitive and Emotional Outcomes from an SMR Training Protocol

Valeska Kouzak

Abstract

This chapter reports cognitive and emotional outcomes from a feasible trial of sensorimotor rhythm (SMR-12–15 Hz) neurofeedback (NFB) in patients with early Parkinson's disease (PD). Eight participants (mean age 65.25 ± 5.75) were distributed into three groups: NFB, sham-NFB (S-NFB), or waitlist (Non-NFB). They completed pre- and post-training assessments, including the Parkinson Disease Cognitive Rating Scale (PD-CRS), Beck Anxiety Inventory (BAI), and Beck Depression Inventory (BDI). Ten NFB sessions targeted SMR at Cz using a respiration-guided protocol. Cognitive outcomes demonstrated that the NFB group showed significant improvement in cognition (PD-CRS total; $p < 0.05$) and in the subcomponents, that is, frontal–subcortical ($p = 0.009$) and cortical–posterior ($p = 0.035$). The S-NFB group showed a significant change in PD-CRS total but not in component subscores. Emotional outcomes demonstrated that the NFB group had significant reductions in anxiety (BAI; $p < 0.05$) and depression (BDI; $p < 0.05$), while controls did not. Consequently, these results indicate that SMR neurofeedback can yield clinically relevant cognitive and affective benefits in early PD.

Keywords: neurofeedback, sensorimotor rhythm, cognition, anxiety, depression, PD-CRS

1. Introduction

Parkinson's disease (PD) is a progressive disorder of the nervous system and the second most common neurodegenerative disease worldwide, affecting about 1–2 individuals per 1,000 in the general population [1]. PD prevalence (the number of existing cases) reflects incidence (the number of new cases) and disease duration, that is, how many years a person lives with the condition. PD incidence is linked to risk and protective factors that may vary across populations according to genetic, socioeconomic, and geographic aspects [2]. Age is the greatest risk factor, followed by exposure to chemicals and environmental pollutants such as pesticides, industrial solvents, and heavy metals. Conversely, smoking is associated with a reduced risk of PD, although a causal relationship remains debated [3].

The most common symptoms that distinguish PD from other progressive disorders are bradykinesia, muscle rigidity, resting tremor, and postural instability [4]. In addition to motor symptoms that reduce quality of life, nonmotor symptoms, such as anosmia, constipation, and neuropsychiatric changes, are also characteristic of the disease [5], as well as neurocognitive loss [6]. This chapter focuses on PD neuropsychiatric and neurocognitive symptoms, applying neurofeedback (NFB) for their regulation.

According to Luria [7], neuropsychology's main goal is to investigate the role of specific brain systems in complex forms of mental activity, that is, to unite cognitive processes (perception, attention, memory, reasoning, emotion, language, planning, and motor control) with neuroscience — how the nervous system is organized and functions [8, 9]. Consequently, in PD, neuronal degeneration across multiple pathways progressively alters the affected individual's mental activity, producing a spectrum of neuropsychological symptoms that should be addressed, beginning with the management of primary motor manifestations.

The loss of dopaminergic neurons in the substantia nigra pars compacta leads to degeneration within the basal ganglia, disrupting thalamic inhibitory circuits and producing hallmark motor manifestations of the disorder, including tremor and freezing. Hence, the neuronal consequence on movement. Physiologically, the cortex maintains movement planning in the premotor and motor regions of the frontal lobe; however, abnormal basal ganglia function impairs the speed of movement initiation, causing actions to remain slow throughout execution [8]. These two examples illustrate the primary neuropsychological impairment in the disorder: motor control.

Consequently, with improved recognition of nonmotor symptoms and a more detailed understanding of pathophysiology, a new view of PD has emerged [10]. Neurocognitive disorders are common in PD; dementia prevalence is 26% at disease onset and longitudinally reaches 78.2% within eight years after diagnosis [6]. Additionally, there is a prevalence of cognitive decline in non-demented patients of 25% [11]. The common pattern of cognitive change in PD is a dysexecutive syndrome, although a range of visuospatial, memory, and language deficits are also observed [12].

Since manifestations vary, it has been proposed that cognitive impairments arise from two partially overlapping syndromes. On one hand, usually primarily, dopaminergic loss in basal circuits produces deficits in attention and executive function; on the other hand, occurring later, it is associated with cholinergic degeneration and cortical posterior involvement, causing impairments in recognition memory and visuospatial skills. This "dual syndrome" model describes domain-specific cognitive deficits: fronto-striatal and/or posterior cortical [13].

PD also presents neuropsychiatric nonmotor symptoms that commonly co-occur as the disease progresses, with anxiety, depression, apathy, and psychosis among the most frequent, affecting most patients at some point during the disease. These symptoms are particularly important because they directly affect patients' quality of life [14].

Depression and anxiety are the two most prevalent neuropsychiatric disorders in PD. Clinically significant depressive symptoms occur in roughly 30%–40% of patients, while anxiety affects about 40%. Symptoms of both conditions can be related to periods "off" medication, which usually parallel motor fluctuations and often respond to antiparkinsonian medication [15]. Both depression and anxiety can precede motor symptoms by several years and are considered prodromal features of the disease [16].

Anxiety, the most common neuropsychiatric symptom among the two mentioned above, affects about 31% of PD patients, according to Kalia and Lang's study [17]. Moreover, recent work suggests that anxiety in PD may be linked to reduced cognitive control over emotional processes [18], becoming an added burden as it can be associated with motor disability and reduced quality of life [19].

Garlovsky et al. identified personality traits, coping style, social support, and disease-related factors as psychosocial predictors of anxiety in PD [20]. Individuals exhibiting avoidant or pessimistic personality traits experience higher levels of anxiety, likely due to a less effective coping style with negative emotional states. In contrast, robust social support and a stable sense of identity appear to confer protective effects.

A systematic review showed that anxiety related to PD is associated with structural and functional changes in the cortico-limbic–striato–thalamo–cortical (CSTC) circuit and in the fear circuit [21]. Anxiety in PD may thus arise from dysregulation among these neural circuits. Besides, shared pathophysiological mechanisms between anxiety and PD may account for their symptom overlap.

The dopaminergic theory indicates that early mesolimbic and mesocortical dopaminergic neurodegeneration in PD is highly associated with anxiety [22]. Depletion of serotonergic neurons in the raphe nuclei [23] increases anxiety symptoms in PD patients [24]. Degeneration of the locus coeruleus, rich in noradrenaline, is responsible for generating physiological anxiety reactions [25]. Consequently, deficits in these neurotransmitter systems contribute to the elevated prevalence of anxiety in PD. Symptom overlap also occurs; that is, anxiety-driven behaviors can mimic PD motor signs (e.g., agitation resembling tremor, restlessness resembling dyskinesia), while PD-related symptoms (muscle tension, fatigue, impaired concentration) may be misinterpreted as anxiety. These overlaps confound differential diagnosis, since symptoms may stem from anxiety, PD, or both [24].

In the case of depression, difficulties in differential diagnosis are also observed, since most of the key features of depression, which are low mood, loss of interest or pleasure (anhedonia), changes in sleep and appetite, loss of libido, psychomotor retardation, impaired memory, and loss of energy, are additionally features that can overlap with the symptoms of PD [15]. Moreover, neurobiological findings suggest that depression in PD is not solely due to serotonergic pathway dysfunction but also involves reduced dopaminergic and noradrenergic innervation of limbic and striatal systems [26].

Consistent with this, depression in PD can be treated with selective serotonin reuptake inhibitors (SSRIs), serotonin–norepinephrine reuptake inhibitors (SNRIs), and dopaminergic agonists [27], alongside antiparkinsonian medications. Denervation of mesolimbic dopaminergic pathways is a key contributor to apathy and depression, accounting for their frequent comorbidity in PD. Evidence shows that dopaminergic agonists can improve depression and apathy in PD patients [28, 29], in line with conceptualizing depression and apathy as hypodopaminergic syndromes in PD. Recent studies also indicate a role for serotonergic pathway degeneration in depression and apathy: a meta-analysis found that 57.2% of apathetic PD patients also had depression, while 42.8% did not, indicating that apathy can be distinct from depression [30]. Apathy severity is primarily related to lesions of the caudate nucleus and orbitofrontal cortex, while depression is linked to the anterior cingulate cortex, which may explain symptom differences [31]. Cholinesterase inhibitors may ameliorate apathy by augmenting cholinergic transmission; however, they do not appear to alter depressive symptoms.

These results suggest that dopaminergic pathways may underlie both apathy and depression, while serotonergic pathways may contribute differently [32]. When anxiety co-occurs with depression in PD, a common scenario, the severity of both is associated with serotonergic pathway alterations as well as the loss of dopaminergic and noradrenergic innervation, confirming the involvement of dopaminergic, serotonergic, and noradrenergic systems in both conditions [32].

Psychosis is also a common neuropsychiatric complication in PD, observed in approximately 26%–60% of patients depending on clinical features, and can range across illusions, hallucinations, and delusions with or without insight. Treatment options are limited because some antipsychotics worsen motor symptoms depending on their pharmacodynamics. The most commonly used agents are quetiapine, clozapine, and pimavanserin, which do not significantly antagonize D2 receptors and therefore do not adversely affect the nigrostriatal dopaminergic motor pathway [33]. Risk factors for psychosis in PD include Rapid Eye Moviment (REM) sleep behavior disorder, older age at disease onset, longer disease duration, depression, antiparkinsonian medication, female sex, dyskinesia, cognitive impairment, and autonomic dysfunction [34]. Widespread gray matter volume loss in parieto–temporo–occipital regions, along with associations between gray matter volume and local expression of serotonergic receptor genes, may be related to psychosis in PD [35].

1.1 Pathophysiology of PD

PD pathophysiology involves degeneration of the nigrostriatal dopaminergic circuit, which underlies the motor changes, and neuronal deposition of α synuclein fibrils as Lewy bodies, affecting brain regions beyond the mesencephalic substantia nigra and involving nondopaminergic neurons [36].

According to Braak's theory [37], PD presents six progressive stages related to α synuclein deposition in the brain. In brief, in stage 1, aggregated α synuclein appears within olfactory structures and the dorsal motor nucleus of the vagus; in stage 2, degeneration follows in the lower portion of the raphe nucleus and the locus coeruleus; in stage 3, the substantia nigra is affected along with the amygdala, pedunculopontine tegmental nucleus, and upper raphe nuclei, among other areas; during stage 4, α synuclein spreads to the hippocampal formation and specific cortical regions; and in the final stages 5 and 6, nearly the entire cortex is involved [38].

Thus, PD patients also show degeneration of multiple other neuronal systems, including the noradrenergic pathway of the locus coeruleus, the dorsal motor nucleus of the vagus, the serotonergic raphe nuclei, the cholinergic basal nucleus of Meynert, the pedunculopontine nucleus, the Edinger-Westphal nucleus, and other brainstem nuclei [39]. Some of these pathways influence the composition of clinical symptoms. It is, therefore, widely accepted that α synuclein propagation in the brain occurs in stages and that lesions in other areas precede degeneration of substantia nigra neurons, affecting glutamatergic, noradrenergic, serotonergic, histaminergic, and cholinergic projections [38].

According to the canonical model [40], alterations in dopaminergic projections to the striatum acting at D1 (excitatory) and D2 (inhibitory) receptors disrupt thalamic signaling. In this framework, dopaminergic denervation produces an imbalance between the direct and indirect pathways, which underlies bradykinesia and rigidity. Neurons in the substantia nigra pars compacta (SNpc) facilitate the D1-mediated direct pathway while suppressing D2-mediated activity in the indirect pathway within distinct populations of medium spiny neurons (MSNs), the principal output neurons of the striatum. MSNs exert inhibitory control over the internal (GPi) and external (GPe) segments of the globus pallidus; the GPi, serving as the principal basal ganglia output nucleus, provides tonic inhibition to the thalamus. Reduced thalamic inhibition then leads to altered excitatory input to the neocortex, completing the basal ganglia–thalamocortical loop and accounting for many of the observed neurophysiological disturbances.

1.2 Neurophysiology of PD

Oscillations in Beta (13–31 Hz) have an important role in movement coordination. They predominate during stability and tonic contractions, decrease immediately before and during movement execution, and show a rebound afterward [41]. Studies support the idea that stopping or withholding undesired behaviors is associated with increased synchronization and coherence of Beta frequency oscillations [42]. Altered Beta oscillations are observed in dorsolateral and frontal regions in PD, which are related to motor processing specifically involved in interrupting movement.

Striatal loss of dopaminergic input induces heightened beta-band oscillatory synchronization across basal ganglia and thalamocortical networks. Coherence in the 15–30 Hz range over the somatosensory area can produce symptom relief in PD [43]. Preclinical models and electrophysiological recordings associate dopaminergic denervation with increased beta-band synchrony throughout basal ganglia and thalamocortical networks. For example, two studies showed that L-dopa treatment reduced beta coherence between the GPi and subthalamic nucleus (STN), and between the STN and supplementary motor area (SMA) during rest or motor tasks [44, 45].

Interhemispheric Beta synchronization may be another electrophysiological feature of PD [36]. Additionally, PD patients undergoing deep brain stimulation (DBS) surgery show Beta oscillations in dorsolateral regions topographically associated with motor areas [46]. Beta band synchronization is thought to promote immutability, stabilizing neural circuits in a low-entropy state and maintaining homeostasis [47]. Elevated Beta synchronization can engage expansive neural assemblies across distributed brain regions, producing predictable, stereotyped spatiotemporal firing patterns.

Excessive Beta synchronization is strongly associated with bradykinesia and rigidity [48], as Beta synchronization facilitates stopping behavior via direct and indirect basal ganglia pathways involving the SNpc and putamen [49]. Other oscillations may explain tremors and dyskinesia [50].

Gamma frequency (35–90 Hz) is fundamental to neuronal computation, arising from inhibitory postsynaptic potentials reverberating in interneuronal networks and between inhibitory and excitatory pyramidal populations to produce recurrent feedback loops [51, 52]. Gamma is associated with motor processing [53].

To this end, we conducted a study with eight patients diagnosed with PD at early stages, recruited through medical clinics and digital media, to test an NFB protocol for training the sensorimotor rhythm (12–15 Hz) that is related to low Beta waves at the sensorimotor cortex. Participants had a mean age of 65.25 years (SD ± 5.75), with six males and two females. All participants were under regular neurological follow-up and met the inclusion and exclusion criteria established for the study.

2. NFB training

2.1 Participants

Participants were randomly allocated into three groups: an experimental NFB group, a sham neurofeedback group (S-NFB), and a non-neurofeedback control group (Non-NFB). The experimental group underwent NF training, the sham group received placebo NF sessions, and the Non-NFB group remained on a waiting list for an equivalent period. After the initial phase, participants in the Non-NFB group were reassigned to either the experimental or sham group for ethical reasons.

The institutional ethics committee approved all procedures, and written informed consent was obtained from every participant.

2.2 NFB protocol

For NFB training, an EEG channel with three electrodes was used, placed on the scalp according to the international 10/20 system, where one was an active electrode positioned at Cz, a reference electrode on the left earlobe, and a ground electrode on the right earlobe. Additionally, two more channels were used to record physiological signals for respiration and heart rate. Ten NFB training sessions were conducted twice weekly.

The Sham-NFB (S-NFB) protocol proceeded as follows: the first session was an NFB training session that was recorded, and the subsequent nine sessions used the recording of the initial training. The control group, which did not undergo NFB (Non-NFB), completed the initial assessment and remained on a waitlist for the training period, approximately one and a half months. Afterward, these subjects were allocated to one of the two groups (NFB or S-NFB).

The NFB device is connected to a computer and uses the BioGraph Infiniti system — Thought Technology, Canada — for signal analysis and NFB.

The initial data collection and training were conducted by the research assistants so that the study remained blind to the investigator, characterizing it as single-blind.

2.3 Cognitive and emotional assessment

2.3.1 PD cognitive rating scale – PD-CRS

The PD-CRS is a cognitive scale developed for patients with PD, given that 23% to 55% of patients exhibit cognitive decline, which is associated with an increased likelihood of progression to PD with subsequent dementia. Because Parkinson's pathophysiology is characterized initially by denervation of dopaminergic circuits and subsequently by denervation of cholinergic circuits in the basal ganglia, cognitive deficits present two patterns: a cortico-frontal profile and a cortico-posterior profile [6]. The scale was recently translated and validated for the Brazilian population and comprises nine tasks divided into immediate verbal memory, confrontation naming, sustained attention, working memory, clock drawing, clock copying, delayed verbal memory, alternating verbal fluency, and action verbal fluency. The visuospatial tasks correspond to cortico-posterior scoring – specifically confrontation naming and clock drawing – while the other tasks assess cortico-frontal functions [53].

2.3.2 Beck depression and anxiety inventories – BDI and BAI

The Beck Depression Inventory (BDI) and Beck Anxiety Inventory (BAI) are symptom-based questionnaires aligned with DSM-IV criteria for each disorder; they were translated and validated for the Brazilian sample by Cunha [54]. In the BDI, respondents select the statement that best describes how they have felt during the past week. In addition to quantifying depressive severity and classifying cases as non-depressed, mild, moderate, or severe according to score, the scale also aims to characterize symptoms and facilitate patient self-awareness in clinical practice. The BAI assesses symptom severity: participants are presented with a list of anxiety-related symptoms and rate each from "did not feel" (0) to "could not bear it" (3), with scores of 1 and 2 indicating milder or moderate intensity; ratings refer to the past week and help patients develop self-perception. In this study, both inventories are used for their practicality and validated performance.

All assessments were conducted before and after the NFB intervention period.

3. Results

For the Anxiety Inventory (BAI), the NFB group had a mean of 8.6 (SD = 3.13) in the first session and 5.4 (SD = 3.61) in the second session. The S-NFB group had a mean of 12.3 (SD = 10.4) in the first session and 6.0 (SD = 5.35) in the second session. In the Non-NFB group, the BAI mean was 5.6 (SD = 3.68) in the first session and 7.3 (SD = 2.35) in the second session (**Table 1**).

For the Depression Inventory (BDI), the NFB group's mean was 11.6 (SD = 3.7) in the first session and 8.2 (SD = 2.7) in the second session. The S-NFB group had a first-session mean of 13.3 (SD = 5.9) and a second-session mean of 10.6 (SD = 7.9). The Non-NFB group's BDI mean was 6.3 (SD = 4.2) in the first session and 9.6 (SD = 3.68) in the second session (**Table 1**).

For the cognitive test (PD-CRS), the NFB group obtained a mean of 83.8 (SD = 17.13) in the first session and 95.7 (SD = 14.7) in the second session. The S-NFB group's first-session mean was 63.0 (SD = 13.9), and the second-session mean was 70.0 (SD = 10.67). The Non-NFB group had a first-session mean of 79.9 (SD = 17.6) and a second-session mean of 81.0 (SD = 20.6) (**Table 1**).

A paired one-tailed t-test analysis was conducted in order to indicate significant differences ($p < 0.05$) between subjects before and after NFB in all conditions for the

Group Subjects	BAI				BDI				PD-CRS			
	Mean 1	SD	Mean 2	SD	Mean 1	SD	Mean 2	SD	Mean 1	SD	Mean 2	SD
NFB	8,6	3,1	5,4	3,6	11,6	3,7	8,2	2,7	83,8	17,13	95,2	14,79
S-NFB	12,3	10,4	6	5,35	13,3	5,9	10,6	7,93	63	13,9	70	10,6
Non-NFB	5,6	3,68	7,3	2,35	6,3	4,1	9,6	3,6	79,6	17,5	81	20,6

Table 1.
Mean and standard deviation of BAI, BDI, and PD-CRS. Where mean 1: mean result of the test before neurofeedback training for all conditions; mean2: mean result of the test after neurofeedback training for all conditions. SD: standard deviation of the mean for each condition; NFB: experimental group; S-NFB: placebo group; non-NFB: waiting-list group.

emotional scales BAI (**Figure 1**) and BDI (**Figure 2**) as well as for cognitive performance PD-CRS in all conditions (**Figure 3**).

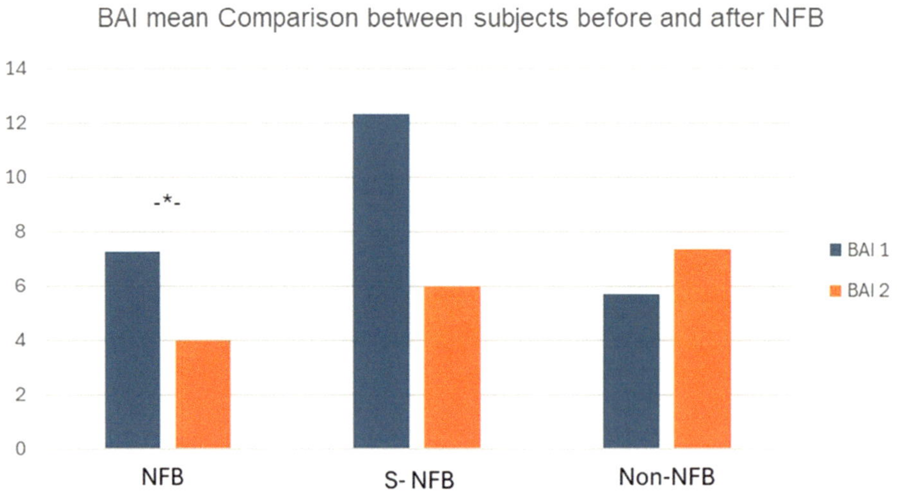

Figure 1.
*The graph in **Figure 1** represents the comparison between the BAI mean scores with-in subjects for the experimental (NFB), placebo control (S-NFB), and non-NFB control group before and after NFB training. Where the blue barr indicate the mean score before the intervention and the orange barr the mean score after the intervention. The asterisk indicates a significant difference* ($p < 0.05$) *in the experimental sample.*

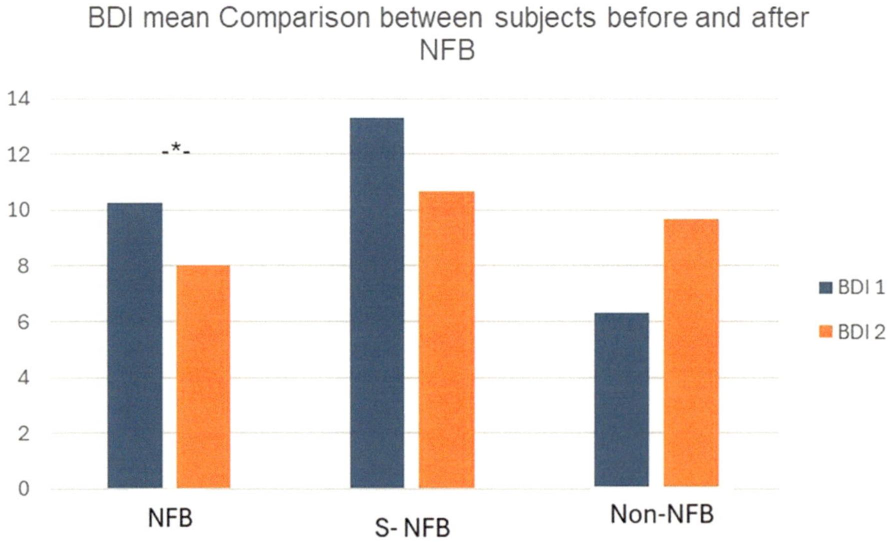

Figure 2.
*The graph in **Figure 2** represents the comparison between the BDI mean scores with-in subjects for the experimental (NFB), placebo control (S-NFB), and non-NFB contol groups before and after NFB training, where the blue barr indicate the mean score before the intervention and the orange barr the mean score after the intervention. The asterisk indicates a significant difference* ($p < 0.05$) *in the experimental sample. Comparison between the mean scores of subjects in the experimental (NFB), placebo control (S-NFB), and non-NFB control groups for the BDI test before and after NFB training. The asterisk indicates a significant difference* ($p < 0.05$) *in the experimental sample.*

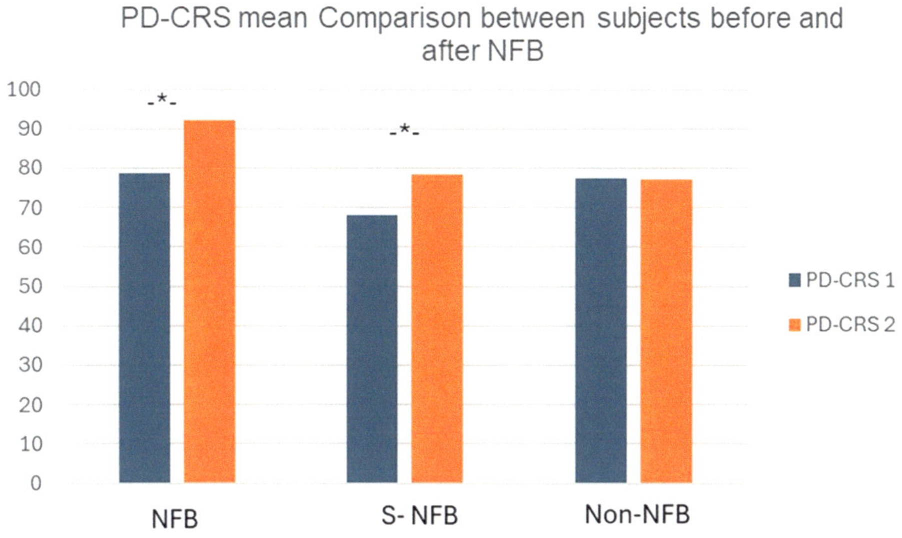

Figure 3.
The graph in ***Figure 3*** *represents the comparison between the PD-CRS mean scores with-in subjects for the experimental (NFB), placebo control (S-NFB), and non-NFB control groups for the PD-CRS test before and after NFB training, where the blue barr indicate the mean score before the intervention and the orange barr indicate the mean score after the intervention. The asterisk indicates a significant difference* ($p < 0.05$) *between the experimental and placebo samples. Comparison between the mean scores of subjects in the experimental (NFB), placebo control (S-NFB), and non-NFB control groups for the PD-CRS test before and after NFB training. The asterisk indicates a significant difference* ($p < 0.05$) *between the experimental and placebo s.*

The results of the t-test between subjects before and after NFB for the experimental group at BAI were $p = 0.0014$, which is significant, and for the S-NFB group ($p = 0.14$) and Non-NFB group ($p = 0.16$), which are not significant. For the t-test between subjects before and after NFB for the experimental group at BDI were $p = 0.04$, which is significant, and for the S-NFB group ($p = 0.14$) and Non-NFB group ($p = 0.14$), which are not significant.

For the PD-CRS, the t-test between subjects before and after NFB for the experimental groups was $p = 0$, and for placebo, $p = 0.03$, which is significant. On the other hand, the Non-NFB group has a $p = 0.45$, which is not significant.

Because significant differences were observed in the cognitive assessment (PD-CRS) for both the experimental and placebo samples, and given the profile of cognitive impairments associated with PD under the dual-syndrome framework, we computed paired t-tests separately for the frontal–subcortical and posterior cortical subscores. Both subscores showed significant improvement in the NFB group: frontal–subcortical, $p = 0.009$; posterior cortical, $p = 0.035$. No significant differences were found in the placebo control group for either subscore, as illustrated in **Figure 4**.

4. Discussion

The present study investigated the effects of EEG-based NFB training on emotional and cognitive aspects in patients with early-stage PD. The findings reveal meaningful effects of NFB on non-motor symptoms, specifically anxiety, depression,

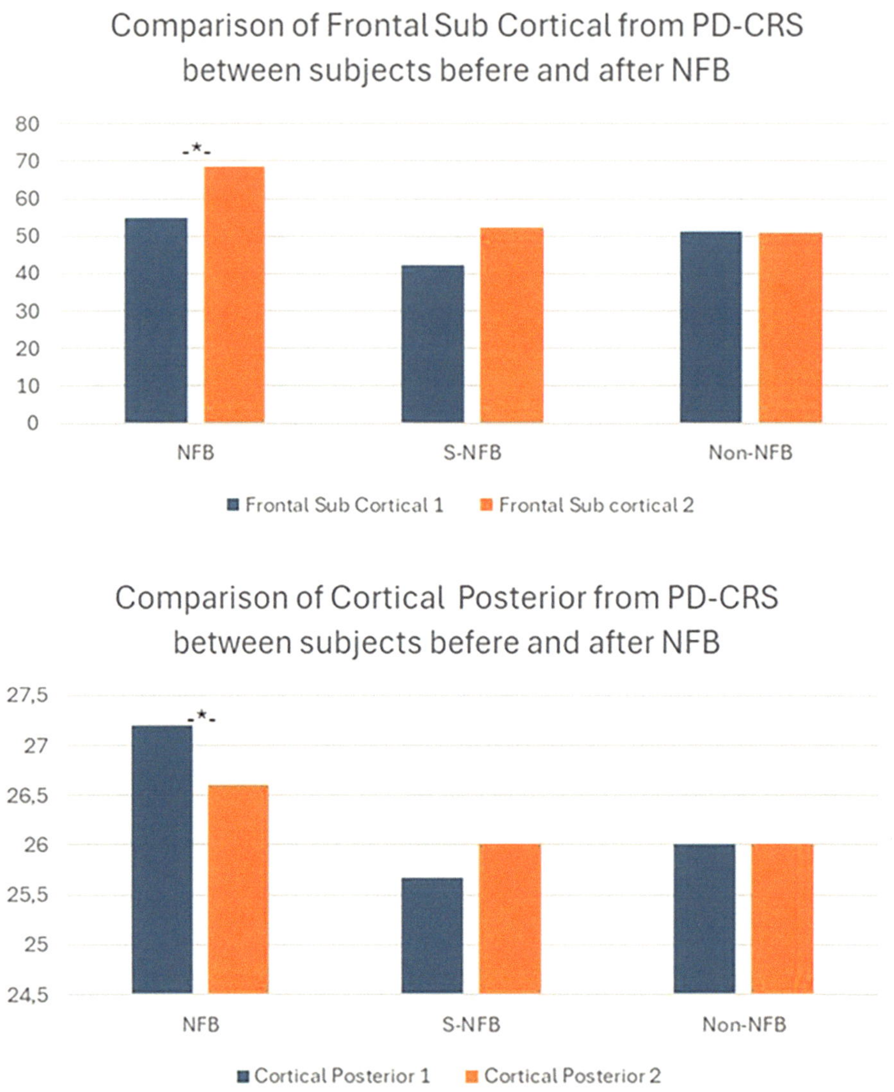

Figure 4.
The graph in ***Figure 4*** *represents the comparison of frontal-subcortical and cortical posterior PD-CRS mean score for experimental group (NFB), placebo group (S-NFB) and waitlist (Non-NFB) before and after NFB training. The blue barr indicate the mean score before intervention and the orange barr indicate the mean score after the intervention. The asterisk indicates a significant difference* (p <*0.05) in the experimental sample for frontal-subcortical and cortical posterior. Comparison of frontal-subcortical PD-CRS results for groups before and after NFB training. The asterisk indicates a significant difference* (p <*0.05) in the experimental sample, as well as a of posterior cortical PD-CRS results for groups before and after NFB training. The asterisk indicates a significant difference* (p <*0.05) in the experimental sample.*

and cognitive performance. Effects of NFB training were observed on behavioral aspects of anxiety ($p < 0.05$), depression ($p < 0.05$), and cognition ($p < 0.05$), which align with other NFB studies showing cognitive improvement in healthy subjects or those with cognitive decline [55] and improvement in emotional symptoms in cases of depression and anxiety [56].

The selection of the sensorimotor rhythm (SMR) protocol for the study is related to the fact that patients with PD tend to increase beta activity in the motor cortex as a compensatory response to dopaminergic loss in the substantia nigra pars compacta of the basal ganglia [36]. However, the results may suggest that distinct neuronal mechanisms are related to motor and non-motor aspects; that is, excessive beta activity in the sensorimotor region appears not only to be related to motor aspects, but its modulation can also affect cognitive aspects [56].

From a neurocognitive perspective, results showed that the difference between tests was statistically significant for the experimental group and also for the placebo group, so the cognitive gain cannot be attributed entirely to NFB. In order to clarify whether there was a gain due to NFB beyond placebo, the analysis was extended to other cognitive outcomes, more specifically outcomes related to the cortical degeneration pattern of the dual syndrome. Only the experimental sample showed significant changes in its results: frontal–subcortical ($p < 0.05$) and posterior cortical ($p < 0.05$).

Hence, significant changes were observed both in the total PD-CRS score and in the sums for frontal–subcortical and posterior cortical domains for patients who underwent NFB training; this can be related to the dual syndrome, in which frontal–subcortical deficits are linked to executive difficulties, working memory, and attention affected by dopaminergic losses in basal circuits, while posterior cortical deficits relate to visuospatial loss affected by cholinergic depletion [57]. In the present study, NFB group patients significantly increased their frontal–subcortical scores and significantly decreased their posterior cortical scores; therefore, they successfully regulated SMR via NFB, which increases attention [13] and, additionally, working memory. Because changes were larger for the frontal–subcortical outcomes, it can be inferred that the training produced changes in dopaminergic pathways in the superior cortical area, which may concurrently influence activity in basal circuits [58].

The PD-CRS result reinforces that NFB is a tool for enhancing cognitive performance, as protocols to improve neurocognitive aspects in healthy adults and older adults have shown good results [59–63]. Likewise, the protocol used in the present study to increase SMR, when applied to healthy older adults, promoted an increase in working memory [64], which is related to attention.

Moreover, the changes in emotion and cognition observed in the experimental group demonstrated that SMR regulation can modify the emotional and cognitive capacity of patients with PD; therefore, NFB is an attractive tool for any disorder involving an imbalance in neural circuits and may indicate a clinically meaningful change [65].

5. Conclusion

This study aimed to test NFB training in PD patients to determine whether it can enhance emotional and cognitive function. The protocol targeted an increase in SMR over the central cortex, based on evidence that PD is associated with beta hyperactivity as a compensatory response to dopaminergic denervation in the basal ganglia.

The findings indicate that NFB training produced emotional improvement by significantly reducing anxiety and depressive symptoms, as measured by the BAI and the BDI. In addition, NFB elicited neurocognitive gains, improving patients' performance on the PD-CRS, particularly in the frontal–subcortical domain.

The significant reduction in anxiety and depressive symptoms observed in the experimental group suggests that neurofeedback training may contribute to emotional regulation in PD patients. Emotional symptoms in PD are highly prevalent and strongly associated with reduced quality of life, often occurring independently of motor symptom severity.

The study has limitations, notably its sample size; therefore, increasing the sample would yield more statistically robust results and expand opportunities for comparative and correlational analyses.

Future research could build on these findings by further exploring relationships between nonmotor symptoms and NFB, using additional scales and neuropsychological tests that assess apathy, executive functions, memory, and attention. Studies could also combine cognitive tasks with emotional components – for example, a working memory task (DMTS) paired with emotionally valenced stimuli (IAPS) – to evaluate both cognitive and emotional domains simultaneously.

The findings underscore the importance of incorporating emotional and cognitive outcomes into intervention studies for PD and support the development of integrative therapeutic models that extend beyond motor symptom management. Future studies with larger samples, extended follow-up, and expanded neuropsychological assessment batteries are warranted to further clarify the mechanisms and durability of these effects.

Acknowledgments

The author would like to thank her team of psychologists: Psy. Wendy Isabel Silvestre da Silva, Psy. Patricia Cardoso da Silva, and Psy. Luisa Wakim Batista, as well as her advisor, PhD. Maria Clotilde Henriques Tavares.

Conflicts of Interest

The author declares no conflicts of interest.

Data availability statement

Data is available upon reasonable request to the corresponding author.

Author details

Valeska Kouzak
Laboratory of Neurosciences and Behavior, Institute of Biological Sciences, University of Brasília, Brasília, Brazil

*Address all correspondence to: valeskakouzak@gmail.com

References

[1] Tysnes OB, Storstein A. Epidemiology of Parkinson's disease. Journal of Neural Transmission. 2017;**124**:901–905. DOI: 10.1007/s00702-017-1686-y

[2] Ben-Shlomo Y, Darweesh S, Llibre-Guerra J, Marras C, San Luciano M, Tanner C. The epidemiology of Parkinson's disease. The Lancet. 2024;**403**(10423):283–292

[3] Dorsey ER, Elbaz A. Global, regional, and national burden of Parkinson's disease, 1990–2016: A systematic analysis for the Global Burden of Disease Study 2016. The Lancet Neurology. 2018;**17**(11):939–953. DOI: 10.1016/S1474-4422(18)30295-3

[4] Abbas MM, Xu Z, Tan LC. Epidemiology of Parkinson's disease—east versus west. Movement Disorders Clinical Practice. 2018;**5**:14–28. DOI: 10.1002/mdc3.12568

[5] Simon DK, Tanner CM, Brundin P. Parkinson disease epidemiology, pathology, genetics, and pathophysiology. Clinics in Geriatric Medicine. 2020;**36**(1):1–12. DOI: 10.1016/j.cger.2019.08.002

[6] Brandão PRP, Munhoz RP, Grippe TC, et al. Cognitive impairment in Parkinson's disease: A clinical and pathophysiological overview. Journal of the Neurological Sciences. 2020;**419**:117177

[7] Luria AR. The Working Memory. London: Basic Books; 1973

[8] Gazzaniga MS, Ivry RB, Mangun GR. Cognitive Neuroscience: The Biology of the Mind. 4th ed. New York: W. W. Norton; 2014

[9] Piccinini JP, Todd DM, Massaro T, et al. Changes in quality of life, cognition and functional status following catheter ablation of atrial fibrillation. Heart 2020;**106**:1919–1926

[10] Jenner P, et al. Parkinson's disease – The debate on the clinical phenomenology, aetiology, pathology and pathogenesis. Journal of Parkinson's Disease. 2013;**3**(s1):1–11. DOI: 10.3233/JPD-130175

[11] Aarsland D, Brønnick K, Larsen JP, Tysnes OB, Alves G. Cognitive impairment in incident, untreated Parkinson disease: The Norwegian ParkWest study. Neurology. 2009;**72**(13):1121–1126. DOI: 10.1212/01.wnl.0000338632.00552.cb

[12] Aarsland D, Andersen K, Larsen JP, Lolk A, Kragh-Sørensen P. Mild cognitive impairment in Parkinson disease: A multicenter pooled analysis. Neurology. 2010;**75**(12):1062–1069. DOI: 10.1212/WNL.0b013e3181f39d0e

[13] Kehagia AA, Barker RA, Robbins TW. Cognitive impairment in Parkinson's disease: The dual syndrome hypothesis. Neurodegenerative Diseases. 2013;**11**(2):79–92. DOI: 10.1159/000341998

[14] Seppi K, Ray Chaudhuri K, Coelho M, et al. Update on treatments for nonmotor symptoms of Parkinson's disease—an evidence-based medicine review. Movement Disorders. 2019;**34**:180–198

[15] Aarsland D, Marsh L, Schrag A. Neuropsychiatric symptoms in Parkinson's disease. Movement

Disorders. 2009;**24**(15):2175–2186. DOI: 10.1002/mds.22589

[16] Postuma RB, Berg D, Stern M, Poewe W, Olanow CW, Oertel W, Obeso J, Marek K, Litvan I, Lang AE, Halliday G, Goetz CG, Gasser T, Dubois B, Chan P, Bloem BR, Adler CH, Deuschl G, et al. MDS clinical diagnostic criteria for Parkinson's disease. Movement Disorders. 2015;**30**(12):1591–1601. DOI: 10.1002/mds.26424

[17] Kalia LV, Lang AE. Parkinson's disease. The Lancet. 2015;**386**(9996):896–912. DOI: 10.1016/S0140-6736(14)61393-3

[18] De Micco R, Satolli S, Siciliano M, et al. Connectivity correlates of anxiety symptoms in drug-naive Parkinson's disease patients. Movement Disorders 2021;**36**:96–105

[19] Carey G, Lopes R, Moonen AJ, et al. Cognitive behavioral therapy for anxiety in Parkinson's disease induces functional brain changes. Journal of Parkinson's Disease 2023;**13**:93–103

[20] Garlovsky JK, Overton PG, Simpson J. Psychological predictors of anxiety and depression in Parkinson's disease: A systematic review. Journal of Clinical Psychology. 2016;**72**(10):979–998

[21] Carey G, Gormez M, de Jong JJA, et al. Neuroimaging of anxiety in Parkinson's disease: A systematic review. Movement Disorders. 2020;**36**:327–339

[22] Péron J, Dondaine T, Le Jeune F, Grandjean D, Vérin M. Emotional processing in Parkinson's disease: A systematic review. Movement Disorders. 2012;**27**(2):186–199. DOI: 10.1002/mds.24025

[23] Chen CPLH, Alder JT, Bray L, et al. Post-synaptic 5-HT 1A and 5-HT 2A receptors are increased in Parkinson's disease neocortex. Annals of the New York Academy of Sciences. 1998;**861**:288–289

[24] Leentjens AF, Dujardin K, Marsh L, et al. Anxiety rating scales in Parkinson's disease: Critique and recommendations. Movement Disorders 2008;**23**:2015–2025

[25] Benarroch EE. Locus coeruleus. Cell and Tissue Research. 2009;**336**(3):573–588

[26] Galts CP, Bettio LE, Jewett DC, et al. Depression in neurodegenerative diseases: Common mechanisms and current treatment options. Neuroscience and Biobehavioral Reviews. 2019;**102**:56–84

[27] Jankovic J, Tan EK. Parkinson's disease: Etiopathogenesis and treatment. Journal of Neurology, Neurosurgery & Psychiatry. 2020;**91**(8):795–808

[28] Mueller C, Rajkumar AP, Wan YM, et al. Assessment and management of neuropsychiatric symptoms in Parkinson's disease. CNS Drugs 2018;**32**:621–635

[29] Castrioto A, Thobois S, Anheim M, et al. Honeymoon study group. A randomized controlled double-blind study of rotigotine on neuropsychiatric symptoms in de novo PD. Npj Parkinson's Disease 2020;**6**:41

[30] Devos D, Moreau C, Maltête D, et al. Rivastigmine in apathetic but dementia and depression-free patients with Parkinson's disease: A double-blind, placebo-controlled, randomised clinical trial. Journal of

Neurology, Neurosurgery & Psychiatry 2014;**85**:668–674

[31] Maillet A, Krack P, Lhommée E, et al. The prominent role of serotonergic degeneration in apathy, anxiety and depression in de novo Parkinson's disease. Brain 2016;**139**:2486–2506

[32] Cong S, Xiang C, Zhang S, Zhang T, Wang H. Prevalence and clinical aspects of depression in Parkinson's disease: A systematic review and meta-analysis of 129 studies. Neuroscience and Biobehavioral Reviews. 2022;**141**:104749. DOI: 10.1016/j.neubiorev.2022.104749

[33] Longardner K, Wright BA, Alakkas A, et al. Assessing the risks of treatment in Parkinson disease psychosis: An in-depth analysis. PLoS One 2023;**18**:e0278262

[34] Chen J, Chen B, Zhao D, et al. Predictors for early onset psychotic symptoms in patientsnewly diagnosed with Parkinson's disease without psychosis at baseline: A 5-year cohort study. CNS Neuroscience & Therapeutics 2024;**30**:e14651

[35] Pisani S, Gunasekera B, Lu Y, et al. Grey matter volume loss in Parkinson's disease psychosis and its relationship with serotonergic gene expession: A meta-analysis. Neuroscience and Biobehavioral Reviews. 2023;**147**:105081

[36] Esmail S, Linden DEJ. Neural networks and neurofeedback in Parkinson's disease. NeuroRegulation. 2014;**1**(3–4):240–272. DOI: 10.15540/nr.1.3-4.240

[37] Braak H, Del Tredici K, Rüb U, de Vos RA, Jansen Steur EN, Braak E. Stages in the development of Parkinson's disease-related pathology. Cell and Tissue Research. 2004;**318**(1):121–134. DOI: 10.1007/s00441-004-0956-9

[38] Paredes-Rodriguez E, Vegas-Suerez S, Morera-Herreraz T, et al. The noradrenergic system in Parkinson's disease. Frontiers in Pharmacology. 2020;**11**:435

[39] Jellinger KA. Neuropathology of Parkinson's Disease. Inflamation in Parkinson's Disease: Scientific and clinical aspects. 2014;25–74

[40] Albin RL, Young AB, Penney JB. The functional anatomy of basal ganglia disorders. Trends in Neurosciences. 1989;**12**:366–375

[41] Alegre M, Lopez-Azcarate J, Obeso I, Wilkinson L, Rodriguez-Oroz MC, Valencia M, Obeso JA. The subthalamic nucleus is involved in successful inhibition in the stop-signal task: A local field potential study in Parkinson's disease. Experimental Neurology. 2013;**239**:1–12. DOI: 10.1016/j.expneurol.2012.08.027

[42] Gilbertson T, Lalo E, Doyle L, Di Lazzaro V, Cioni B, Brown P. Existing motor state is favored at the expense of new movement during 13–35 Hz oscillatory synchrony in the human corticospinal system. The Journal of Neuroscience. 2005;**25**:7771–7779

[43] Marsden JF, Limousin-Dowsey P, Ashby P, Pollak P, Brown P. Subthalamic nucleus, sensorimotor cortex and muscle interrelationships in Parkinson's disease. Brain. 2001;**124**:378–388

[44] Brown P, Oliviero A, Mazzone P, et al. Dopamine dependency of oscillations between subthalamic nucleus and pallidum in Parkinson's

disease. The Journal of Neuroscience 2001;**21**:1033–1038

[45] Cassidy M, Mazzone P, Oliviero A, et al. Movement-related changes in synchronization in the human basal ganglia. Brain 2002;**125**:1235–1246

[46] Romanelli P, Esposito V, Schaal DW, Heit G. Somatotopy in the basal ganglia: Experimental and clinical evidence for segregated sensorimotor channels. Brain Research Reviews. 2005;**48**:112–128

[47] Engel AK, Fries P. Beta-band oscillations—signalling the status quo? Current Opinion in Neurobiology. 2010;**20**:156–165. DOI: 10.1016/j.conb.2010.02.015

[48] Zaidel A, Spivak A, Grieb B, Bergman H, & Israel Z. Subthalamic span of β oscillations predicts deep brain stimulation efficacy for patients with Parkinson's disease. Brain. 2010;**133** (7):2007–2021

[49] Mehler DMA. Turning markers into targets – Scoping neural circuits for motor neurofeedback training in Parkinson's disease. Brain-Apparatus Communication: A Journal of Bacomics. 2022;**1**(1):1–27. DOI: 10.1080/27706710.2022.2061300

[50] Richter U, Halje P, Petersson P. Mechanisms underlying cortical resonant states: Implications for levodopa-induced dyskinesia. Revneuro. 2013;**24**:415–429. DOI: 10.1515/revneuro-2013-0018

[51] Fries P. Neuronal gamma-band synchronization as a fundamental process in cortical computation. Annual Review of Neuroscience. 2009;**32**:209–224. DOI: 10.1146/annurev.neuro.051508.135603

[52] Buzsáki G, Wang XJ. Mechanisms of gamma oscillations. Annual Review of Neuroscience. 2012;**35**:203–225. DOI: 10.1146/annurev-neuro-062111-150444

[53] Jenkinson N, Kuhn AA, Brown P. Gamma oscillations in the human basal ganglia. Experimental Neurology. 2013;**245**:72–76. DOI: 10.1016/j.expneurol.2012.07.005

[54] Brandão PRP, Pereira DA, Grippe TC, Bispo DDC, Maluf FB, Yunes MP, Nunes Filho G, Alves CHL, Pagonabarraga J, Kulisevsky J, da Costa AML, Serafim CFDV, Ferreira ACDB, Bastos AMM, Belchior ACF, de Almeida BLC, de Almeida E Castro BM, Matos MS, de Matos RC, Rios GA, Carneiro LO, da Mota BCC, Castro LEDR, Rocha VLS, Tavares MCH, Cardoso F. Parkinson's Disease-Cognitive Rating Scale (PD-CRS): Normative data and mild cognitive impairment assessment in Brazil. Movement Disorders Clinical Practice. 2023;**10**(3):452–465. DOI: 10.1002/mdc3.13657

[55] Trambaiolli LR, Cassani R, Mehler DN, Falk T. Neurofeedback and the aging brain: A systematic review of training protocols for dementia and mild cognitive impairment. Frontiers in Aging Neuroscience. 2021;**13**:682683. DOI: 10.3389/fnagi.2021.682683

[56] Esmail S, Linden DEJ. Emotion regulation networks and neurofeedback in depression. Cognitive Science. 2011;**6**(2):101

[57] Shi Z, Ding L, Han X, Jiang B, Zhang J, Suo D, Yan T. Multimodal biofeedback for Parkinson's disease motor and nonmotor symptoms. Brain Science Advances. 2023;**9** (2):136–154

[58] Arns M, Heinrich H, Strehl U. Evaluation of neurofeedback in ADHD: The long and winding road. Biological Psychology. 2014;**95**:108–115. DOI: 10.1016/j.biopsycho.2013.11.013

[59] Subramanian L, Hindle JV, Johnston S, Roberts MV, Husain M, Goebel R, Linden D. Real-time functional magnetic resonance imaging neurofeedback for treatment of Parkinson's disease. The Journal of Neuroscience. 2011;**31**(45):16309–16317

[60] Vernon D, Egner T, Cooper N, Compton T, Neilands C, Sheri A, Gruzelier J. The effects of training distinct neurofeedback protocols aspects of cognitive performance. International Journal of Psychophysiology. 2003;**47**(1):75–85

[61] Gruzelier JH. A theory of alpha/theta neurofeedback, creative performance enhancement, long distance functional connectivity and psychological integration. Cognitive Processing. 2008;**10**(suppl 1):101–109

[62] Gruzelier JH. EEG-neurofeedback for optimising performance. I: A review of cognitive and affective outcome in healthy participants. Neuroscience and Biobehavioral Reviews. 2014;**44**:124–141. DOI: 10.1016/j.neubiorev.2013.09.015

[63] LeComte G, Juhel J. The effects of neurofeedback training on memory performance in elderly subjects. Psychology. 2011;**2**(8):846–852

[64] Hosseini SH, Pritchard-Berman M, Sosa N, Ceja A, Kesler SR. Task-based neurofeedback training: A novel approach toward training executive functions. Neuroimage. 2016;**134**:153–159

[65] da Paz Vk C, Garcia A, da Paz Neto A C, Tomaz C. SMR neurofeedback facilitates working memory performance in healthy older adults: A behavior and EEG study. Frontiers in Behavioral Neuroscience. 2018;**12**:321. DOI: 10.3389/fnbeh.2018.00321

Chapter 4

Advances in Deep Brain Stimulation for Parkinson's Disease: Clinical Foundations, Procedural Strategies and Anesthetic Considerations

Nicholas Sookhoo, Ivy Zhou and Jie Zhou

Abstract

Deep brain stimulation (DBS) has become a well-established option for patients with Parkinson's disease (PD) whose motor symptoms are no longer well-controlled with medication alone. As DBS has been used more widely, it has become clear that good outcomes depend on more than just the hardware. Patient selection, surgical planning, and careful perioperative management all play a role. This chapter provides an overview of DBS in PD, bringing together what we know about disease neurobiology, neurosurgery, and anesthetic care. We review the basal ganglia–thalamocortical circuits involved in motor dysfunction and describe how neuromodulation of these pathways can lead to meaningful symptom improvement. We also discuss key considerations for patient selection and target choice, along with current procedural approaches, including awake and asleep implantation, stereotactic targeting, and the use of microelectrode recording. Specific attention is given to perioperative anesthetic management, which can shape patient safety and comfort, preserve intraoperative neurophysiologic assessment, and support accurate lead placement. Topics discussed include sedation strategies, airway and hemodynamic challenges, medication interactions, and postoperative recovery in a patient population that is particularly vulnerable to autonomic and neuropsychiatric complications. Postoperative programming, recognition of complications, and emerging innovations such as adaptive DBS systems are also reviewed. This chapter aims to highlight the importance of coordinated multidisciplinary care in optimizing outcomes for patients with PD undergoing DBS.

Keywords: deep brain stimulation, perioperative anesthetic management, Parkinson's disease, motor symptom modulation, functional neurosurgery

1. Introduction

Parkinson's disease (PD) is a progressive neurodegenerative condition marked by a mix of motor and non-motor symptoms that unfold over time and can significantly affect quality of life [1]. Early on, many patients do well with dopaminergic medications. Over the long term, treatment can be complicated by motor fluctuations, dyskinesias, and less consistent symptom control [2, 3]. As the disease advances, medication adjustments stop providing reliable relief, highlighting the limits of pharmacologic therapy in advanced PD [4].

Deep brain stimulation (DBS) is a well-established option for patients whose symptoms are no longer adequately controlled with medication. By modulating abnormal activity within the basal ganglia–thalamocortical network, DBS can lead to sustained improvements in motor symptoms, lower medication requirements, and better functional outcomes [5–7]. Over the past few decades, advances in surgical techniques, neuroimaging, and device technology have broadened the use of DBS and improved its safety and effectiveness [8]. Still, successful therapy depends on more than precise lead placement and requires careful coordination across specialties.

Care for patients undergoing DBS is multidisciplinary. Neurologists, neurosurgeons, psychiatrists, and anesthesiologists all play key roles in delivering DBS safely and effectively [9]. Anesthetic management is especially important, as decisions about sedation, airway management, hemodynamic control, and medication use can directly influence intraoperative neurophysiology, patient cooperation, and postoperative recovery [10, 11]. Even so, anesthesia has often received less attention than other factors when DBS outcomes are discussed.

In this chapter, we present an overview of DBS for PD, bringing together neurobiological foundations, patient selection, functional neurosurgical principles, and perioperative anesthetic considerations. We review contemporary procedural approaches, postoperative programming, complication recognition, and emerging innovations, with particular emphasis on the anesthetic perspective – how sedation choices, physiological management, and medication strategies interact with neurophysiological mapping, targeting accuracy, and perioperative recovery within a coordinated, multidisciplinary workflow.

2. Neurobiological basis of deep brain stimulation in Parkinson's disease

PD is understood as a disorder of dysfunctional motor circuits. The hallmark features of bradykinesia, rigidity, tremor, and postural instability arise due to progressive disruption of the basal ganglia–thalamocortical networks that normally control movement initiation, scaling, and coordination [12–14]. Seeing PD through this circuit-based lens helps explain why DBS works: it targets abnormal network activity instead of simply trying to replace missing neurotransmitter signaling.

Under normal conditions, motor output is shaped by parallel, tightly regulated pathways connecting the cerebral cortex, basal ganglia, thalamus, and motor cortex. Dopaminergic input from the substantia nigra pars compacta plays a key role in maintaining balance within this system by promoting activity in the direct pathway while dampening the indirect pathway [15, 16]. In PD, the loss of dopaminergic neurons disrupts this balance. The result is excessive inhibitory output from the globus pallidus internus (GPi) and substantia nigra pars reticulata to the thalamus, which leads to reduced excitatory drive to the motor cortex [17]. Clinically, this translates into difficulty initiating movement, slower movements, and reduced movement amplitude.

In addition to changes in overall firing rates, PD is also recognized as a disorder of faulty network dynamics. Dopamine depletion promotes pathological synchronization and exaggerated oscillatory activity within basal ganglia circuits, particularly in the beta frequency range [18–20]. These abnormal oscillations can interfere with normal information processing and motor flexibility and are closely linked to the severity of bradykinesia and rigidity in many patients [20, 21]. Beta activity fluctuates with dopaminergic medication states, offering a window into both symptom expression and treatment response; however, beta is a dominant – but not exclusive – marker, and its relationship to clinical state can vary across individuals, PD phenotypes, and recording targets. As the disease progresses, compensatory mechanisms lose effectiveness, and medication alone often fails to restore more normal network behavior.

DBS targets these abnormalities through neuromodulation rather than permanent lesioning. High-frequency stimulation of key motor circuit nodes, such as the subthalamic nucleus (STN) or globus pallidus internus, alters pathological firing patterns and disrupts abnormal synchronization [5, 22, 23]. While the exact mechanisms of DBS are not fully understood, evidence suggests that stimulation suppresses pathological oscillations, regularizes neuronal output, and helps reestablish more physiologic signaling [21, 24, 25]. The effects of DBS extend beyond the immediate stimulation site because it influences motor networks through both orthodromic and antidromic pathways.

This circuit-based framework helps explain the clinical benefits of DBS, including improved motor function, reduced medication-related complications, and more consistent symptom control in advanced PD. It also grounds the biologic foundation for decisions around target selection, stimulation programming, and procedural strategy, directly linking underlying neurobiology to functional neurosurgery and perioperative management.

3. Patient selection and preoperative evaluation

Choosing the right patients is one of the most important factors in achieving good outcomes with DBS for PD. DBS does not slow or reverse disease progression; instead, it is a symptomatic therapy aimed at treating motor complications that are no longer well-controlled with medication. For that reason, careful preoperative evaluation is critical to identify patients who are most likely to benefit while limiting neurologic, psychiatric, and perioperative risks.

Currently, DBS is considered for patients with idiopathic PD who have disabling motor fluctuations, dyskinesias, or medication-refractory tremor despite optimized pharmacologic therapy [26–28]. A strong and sustained response to levodopa remains one of the best predictors of postoperative motor improvement, as DBS tends to stabilize the benefits of dopaminergic therapy rather than improve symptoms that are poorly dopamine-responsive [27, 29]. Patients whose symptoms are dominated by bradykinesia, rigidity, and tremor usually experience greater benefit than those with prominent axial features, such as gait freezing, postural instability, or speech dysfunction, which respond less reliably to stimulation [29, 30].

Several patient-specific factors are associated with more favorable outcomes, some of which include younger age at surgery, shorter disease duration, preserved cognitive function, and the absence of significant psychiatric comorbidity [26, 31, 32]. From a perioperative standpoint, stable cardiovascular status, limited autonomic dysfunction, and the ability to tolerate prolonged operative positioning are also important, particularly when awake implantation is planned. These considerations highlight the importance of involving anesthesia early in the evaluation process and not solely as an intraoperative concern.

Certain conditions represent absolute or relative contraindications to DBS. Patients with atypical or secondary parkinsonian syndromes, such as multiple system atrophy or progressive supranuclear palsy, generally have poor and often short-lived responses to neuromodulation and are not appropriate candidates [33]. Severe dementia is widely considered a contraindication because of the risk of postoperative cognitive decline and limited functional gain [34]. Other high-risk features include active psychosis, severe depression, or significant medical comorbidities that increase surgical or anesthetic risk, as well as marked autonomic instability [31, 35]. Advanced age alone is not an absolute contraindication, but older patients may face higher rates of cognitive, psychiatric, and perioperative complications, making individualized risk-benefit assessment essential [32].

Comprehensive neuropsychological and psychiatric evaluation is a core component of DBS candidacy assessment. Evaluation includes global cognition, executive function, memory, attention, and visuospatial skills, which identify patients at increased risk for postoperative cognitive decline [34, 36]. Psychiatric screening is equally important, as mood disorders, impulse control disorders, and behavioral changes can worsen after DBS or be influenced by target selection and stimulation settings [35, 37]. These evaluations also help guide preoperative counseling, helping set realistic postoperative expectations.

Neuroimaging plays a complementary role in preoperative evaluation, serving both diagnostic and planning purposes. Structural magnetic resonance imaging (MRI) is used to exclude alternative diagnoses, assess cerebrovascular disease or significant cortical atrophy, and define anatomic targets for stereotactic planning [38]. More advanced imaging modalities, like diffusion-based tractography and connectomic analyses, are being further explored to refine target selection and predict outcomes, but their routine clinical use is still evolving [39].

The perioperative assessment also includes a clear plan for antithrombotic management, as intracranial hemorrhage remains an uncommon but potentially devastating complication of DBS implantation. Patients taking antiplatelet agents or anticoagulants should be reviewed collaboratively by neurosurgery, anesthesia, and the prescribing clinician to balance bleeding risk against thromboembolic risk. A safe approach involves confirming the indication and urgency of antithrombotic therapy, assessing patient-specific thrombotic risk, determining whether temporary interruption or bridging is appropriate, and defining laboratory targets and timing for postoperative resumption. Because protocols vary by institution and procedural strategy, explicit documentation and communication with the operative team are essential.

Optimal patient selection for DBS is best achieved through collaborative decision-making among movement disorder neurologists, functional neurosurgeons, anesthesiologists, and psychiatrists. This allows for a balanced assessment of expected motor benefit against neurologic, psychiatric, and perioperative risks. With an integrated approach, both short- and long-term outcomes for patients undergoing DBS are maximized.

4. Targets and functional neurosurgery considerations

The positive health outcomes of DBS in PD depend on more than just choosing the right patient. Thoughtful target selection and precise surgical execution are just as important. DBS targets are selected to modulate dysfunctional nodes within the basal ganglia–thalamocortical circuits, with the aim of improving motor symptoms while limiting unwanted side effects. Among the available options, the STN and the GPi have become the primary targets in PD [40–42].

Stimulation of the STN is associated with strong improvement in bradykinesia, rigidity, and tremor, and often allows for a meaningful reduction in dopaminergic medications [41, 43]. This medication-sparing effect can be particularly helpful for patients affected by medication-related dyskinesias or motor fluctuations. At the same time, STN DBS has been linked to a higher risk of stimulation-related cognitive and neuropsychiatric side effects in some patients, particularly those with preexisting vulnerabilities [44, 45]. These risks highlight the need for careful neuropsychological evaluation and multidisciplinary discussion when considering the STN as a target.

GPi DBS offers comparable improvement in core motor symptoms but with a different side effect profile. Here, stimulation is particularly effective for controlling dyskinesias and is often preferred when medication reduction is not a primary goal or when involuntary movements dominate the clinical picture [42, 46]. Compared with STN DBS, GPi DBS may carry a lower risk of cognitive or mood-related adverse effects, making it a more suitable option for patients with borderline cognitive function or underlying psychiatric disease [45, 47]. Choosing between STN and GPi, therefore, involves more than symptom severity alone and should consider disease stage, medication tolerance, cognitive status, and overall risk.

In some cases, symptom-dominant presentations may prompt consideration of alternative targets. Patients with tremor-dominant PD that is refractory to medication may benefit from stimulation of the ventral intermediate nucleus (VIM) of the thalamus, particularly when tremor is the main disabling feature [48]. While VIM DBS can provide excellent tremor control, it has little effect on other parkinsonian motor symptoms and is generally reserved for carefully selected patients rather than those with more generalized disease [49]. Other targets, such as the pedunculopontine nucleus, have been explored for gait and postural instability, but results have been mixed, and these approaches remain investigational [50].

Regardless of the target, core functional neurosurgical principles are central to successful DBS implantation. Accurate localization, careful trajectory planning, and avoidance of vascular brain structures are critical to reducing surgical risk and optimizing outcomes [51]. Intraoperative tools like microelectrode recording (MER) and test stimulation are used to refine target localization by assessing physiological responses and stimulation-related side effects in real time. These techniques place specific demands on anesthetic management, since sedative agents and physiological changes can alter neuronal firing patterns and patient responsiveness.

Advances in imaging with high-resolution MRI, tractography, and connectomic approaches further refine targeting by allowing more detailed visualization of patient-specific anatomy and network connectivity [39, 52]. Concurrently, technological innovations such as directional leads and current steering have expanded the ability to shape stimulation fields after implantation, potentially improving efficacy while reducing adverse effects [53]. These developments reinforce the idea that DBS is not a one-time intervention but a dynamic therapy that integrates neurobiology, surgical precision, and postoperative programming. With this information, it is understood that target selection and surgical strategy must be individualized, balancing expected motor benefit against cognitive, psychiatric, and perioperative risk.

5. Procedural strategies for DBS implantation

Successful DBS implantation relies on precise stereotactic targeting, disciplined surgical workflows, and thoughtful use of neurophysiologic and imaging data. The clinical impact of DBS hinges on millimeter-level accuracy during electrode placement; because of this, procedural strategy sits right at the intersection of neurobiology, functional neurosurgery, and perioperative management.

Stereotactic targeting begins with high-resolution preoperative imaging to define patient-specific anatomy and establish target coordinates within deep brain structures. MRI and computerized tomography (CT) are used to visualize the STN, GPi, and nearby structures while accounting for individual anatomic variation [54, 55]. Target coordinates are then refined using standardized atlases, direct visualization when possible, and careful trajectory planning to reduce vascular risk and avoid key cortical and subcortical regions [51, 56]. These steps form the backbone of DBS implantation and are essential whether the procedure is performed awake or asleep.

Both awake and asleep approaches are widely used in current practice, with technique selection shaped by institutional preference and patient factors. Awake DBS has traditionally allowed for intraoperative neurologic assessment and MER to confirm target localization based on characteristic firing patterns [57]. Test stimulation can be performed during the procedure to evaluate immediate motor benefit and identify stimulation-related side effects, offering real-time feedback that may help fine-tune lead placement. However, awake surgery places real demands on patients, requiring cooperation, prolonged immobility, and careful anesthetic management to preserve neurophysiologic signals while maintaining comfort.

Asleep DBS, performed under general anesthesia, has become more common as imaging accuracy and intraoperative navigation have improved. Image-guided asleep DBS removes the need for patient participation during lead placement and may reduce perioperative stress, particularly for patients with anxiety, severe tremor, or limited ability to tolerate awake surgery [58, 59]. Comparative studies suggest that, in experienced centers with optimized imaging and targeting workflows, asleep DBS can achieve motor outcomes comparable to awake approaches [60]. Because results may vary with factors such as imaging quality, institutional experience, and the role of intraoperative neurophysiology (including MER), technique selection is best individualized. In practice, the choice between awake and asleep techniques reflects a balance between physiologic confirmation, patient tolerance, and anesthetic priorities.

DBS implantation can be performed as a staged procedure or as a single-session operation, depending on institutional workflow and patient-specific considerations. In staged approaches, intracranial lead placement is performed first, followed later by pulse generator implantation and lead extension tunneling. This sequencing allows detailed neurologic assessment during lead placement while reserving generator implantation for a shorter, more conventional anesthetic. It also creates two distinct perioperative periods with different priorities: the cranial stage emphasizes hemodynamic stability and hemorrhage avoidance, while the chest or pocket stage focuses on infection prevention, analgesia, and minimizing device-related interference. Clearly outlining the workflow and anesthesia plan for each stage helps improve team coordination and sets clearer expectations for patients and caregivers.

MER has played a central role in DBS implantation, particularly for targeting the STN. MER allows surgeons to map neuronal firing patterns along the planned trajectory and identify physiologic signatures that define target boundaries [57, 61]. This method does have drawbacks, as multiple microelectrode passes may increase hemorrhage risk, and recordings are sensitive to anesthetic agents, physiologic fluctuations, and patient movement [62, 63]. As imaging techniques have advanced, some centers have reduced their reliance on MER, especially in asleep DBS, instead favoring image-based targeting strategies.

Ongoing technological advances continue to influence how DBS procedures are performed. Improvements in MRI resolution, susceptibility-weighted imaging, and tractography have enhanced visualization of deep brain targets and their connected networks [52, 64]. More recently, hardware innovations like segmented directional leads now allow postoperative current steering, which gives clinicians more flexibility to shape stimulation fields and manage side effects without moving electrodes [53, 65]. These developments have shifted some emphasis away from intraoperative precision alone toward a broader therapeutic window that extends into postoperative programming.

Taken together, these considerations demonstrate that DBS implantation is not a one-size-fits-all operation. It is a tailored intervention that integrates patient anatomy, symptom profile, surgical dogma, and perioperative planning. Understanding the strengths and limitations of each procedural approach is key to optimizing outcomes and provides important context for the anesthetic strategies discussed in the following section.

6. Perioperative anesthetic management

Perioperative anesthetic management plays an important role in the safety and procedural success of DBS surgery. Like many neurosurgical procedures, DBS demands that anesthetic strategies strike a careful balance between patient comfort and safety, as well as the preservation of neurophysiologic signals, hemodynamic stability, and neurologic assessment. These priorities are complicated by the underlying pathophysiology of PD, including autonomic dysfunction, dependence on dopaminergic medications, and a heightened vulnerability to cognitive and psychiatric disturbances.

The overarching anesthetic goals in DBS surgery include maintaining patient cooperation when needed, minimizing interference with neuronal firing patterns and microelectrode recordings, ensuring stable cerebral perfusion, and avoiding drug interactions that may worsen motor or non-motor symptoms [10, 66]. As a result, anesthetic planning is individualized, considering the surgical approach, target selection, and each patient's neurologic and medical profile.

For awake DBS procedures, sedation is typically used to provide anxiolysis and comfort while preserving responsiveness and neurophysiologic integrity. Short-acting agents, such as dexmedetomidine, low-dose propofol, or carefully titrated opioids, are commonly employed to achieve an adequate level of sedation [67–69]. Dexmedetomidine is frequently favored because it causes minimal respiratory depression and has relatively limited effects on neuronal firing at low doses. Still, excessive sedation can suppress tremor and alter microelectrode recordings, so dosing needs to be handled carefully [50]. Ongoing communication between the anesthesia and surgical teams is critical, as sedation depth often needs to be adjusted throughout different phases of the procedure.

Asleep DBS, performed under general anesthesia, avoids the need for patient participation during lead placement and may be better tolerated by patients with significant anxiety, severe tremor, or limited ability to cooperate during awake surgery. That said, general anesthetic agents can influence neuronal activity and local field potentials, which may affect targeting accuracy when MER is used [51, 63]. For this reason, asleep DBS relies heavily on image-guided targeting and intraoperative imaging confirmation. Anesthetic techniques in this setting typically prioritize hemodynamic stability, smooth and timely emergence, and avoidance of agents that increase the risk of hypotension or postoperative confusion.

Airway management presents unique challenges in DBS surgery, regardless of the anesthetic approach. During awake procedures, maintaining a patent airway can be difficult in patients immobilized in stereotactic frames, where access is limited and rescue options are constrained [70]. In asleep DBS, airway instrumentation must account for restricted head and neck positioning, frame placement, and limited access once surgery is underway. Careful preoperative assessment, a clear airway plan, and well-defined contingency strategies are essential. In addition, patient positioning might be prolonged and uncomfortable, increasing the risk of pressure-related injuries.

Because DBS involves permanently implanted intracranial leads and pulse generators, perioperative planning must also address device-related operating room safety and the risk of electromagnetic interference. When electrocautery is required, most often during lead tunneling or generator pocket creation, bipolar cautery is generally preferred. If monopolar cautery cannot be avoided, it should be used in short, intermittent bursts at the lowest effective settings, with grounding pad placement designed to direct current away from intracranial leads and the pulse generator. Stimulation is commonly turned off during electrocautery, with postoperative reactivation and functional checks performed according to institutional protocols. External defibrillation or cardioversion can be performed when clinically necessary, but pad placement should minimize current flow across the device, and post-event device interrogation should be considered. MRI and other sources of electromagnetic exposure require strict adherence to manufacturer guidelines, which vary by system, lead configuration, and scanner parameters. Beyond the index surgery, anesthesiologists should recognize that patients with DBS frequently present for unrelated procedures, making advance planning around device status, electrocardiographic artifacts, avoidance of diathermy or therapeutic ultrasound near implanted components, and coordination with neurology or neurosurgery teams especially important.

Hemodynamic management is particularly important in patients with PD, who often have autonomic dysfunction, manifesting as orthostatic hypotension, labile blood pressures, and impaired heart rate variability [52]. Intraoperative hypotension may compromise cerebral perfusion and worsen neurologic outcomes, while hypertension increases the risk of intracranial hemorrhage during lead placement [71]. Anesthetic care, therefore, emphasizes tight blood pressure control, cautious fluid administration, and judicious use of vasoactive medications.

Medication management is another critical aspect of perioperative care. Abrupt interruption of dopaminergic therapy can lead to worsening rigidity and akinesia, and, in rare cases, parkinsonism–hyperpyrexia syndrome [53]. Whenever possible, antiparkinsonian medications should be continued throughout the perioperative period, with careful attention to interactions with anesthetic agents, sedatives, and antiemetics. Dopamine antagonists, including metoclopramide and certain antipsychotics, should be avoided due to the risk of symptom exacerbation [72].

Maintaining medication continuity requires advance planning, especially in patients who are NPO or have delayed gastric emptying, both of which are common in PD. When feasible, surgical timing should be coordinated to minimize missed doses, and alternative routes of administration should be arranged ahead of time if oral therapy must be interrupted. Antiemetic choice also matters, as dopamine antagonists can worsen parkinsonian symptoms and should be avoided, while serotonin antagonists and corticosteroids are often safer options. Clear guidance on the timing of the last preoperative dose, the earliest safe postoperative resumption, and medications to avoid helps reduce the risk of rigidity, autonomic instability, and postoperative confusion.

In the next section, we delve into postoperative recovery after DBS surgery, which requires close monitoring for neurologic, cognitive, and psychiatric complications. Patients with PD are at increased risk for delirium, confusion, and hallucinations, particularly in the setting of older age, baseline cognitive impairment, or polypharmacy [73, 74]. Pain management should be balanced to avoid excessive sedation, and early resumption of dopaminergic medications is essential.

7. Postoperative management and programming

Postoperative management after DBS surgery marks the shift from a technically successful procedure to a lasting clinical benefit. Accurate lead placement is necessary, but long-term outcomes depend just as much on close postoperative monitoring and coordinated follow-up. The early postoperative period is especially important, since patients with PD are vulnerable to neurologic, cognitive, and psychiatric complications that can shape both recovery and future programming decisions.

Immediate postoperative care centers on neurologic observation, hemodynamic stability, and early detection of surgical complications. Patients are monitored closely for changes in mental status, new focal neurologic deficits, headache, or signs of intracranial hemorrhage or infection [75, 76]. Postoperative imaging is also commonly obtained to confirm lead position. Timely resumption of antiparkinsonian medications is another essential treatment aspect to prevent worsening rigidity, akinesia, or autonomic instability. Pain control should also be monitored, avoiding excessive sedation that can cloud neurologic assessment, particularly in older patients or those with baseline cognitive impairment.

Standardized postoperative pathways help streamline care and improve early recognition of complications. Many centers obtain early imaging to verify lead placement and screen for hemorrhage, especially when neurologic exams are limited by sedation, preexisting deficits, or delirium risk. Beyond routine neurologic checks, clinicians exhibit a low threshold for urgent imaging in the presence of new focal deficits, severe headache, persistent nausea or vomiting, altered mental status, or delayed emergence from anesthesia. Practical measures, such as early mobilization, careful blood pressure control, and consistent access to scheduled dopaminergic medications, also support recovery and reduce downstream challenges during programming.

Early postoperative motor improvement does not always reflect true stimulation benefit. In many cases, it represents a transient "microlesion effect" from lead passage and local tissue disruption. Recognizing this phenomenon helps avoid premature judgments about efficacy, prevents overly aggressive medication reductions, and supports delaying initial programming until postoperative edema resolves. Waiting also improves the interpretability of programming responses and reduces the risk of attributing short-lived improvements to stimulation settings.

The timing of initial DBS programming varies by center but most commonly occurs several weeks after surgery, once microlesion effects and postoperative edema have subsided [77]. Programming too early can complicate parameter optimization, as early symptom changes may not reflect true stimulation effects. As a result, programming is typically approached as a gradual, iterative process that balances symptom relief against stimulation-related side effects.

DBS programming involves systematic adjustment of parameters such as contact selection, amplitude, pulse width, and frequency. These variables interact and shape the volume of tissue activated, generating both therapeutic benefits and adverse effects [78, 79]. Programming strategies are guided by target choice, lead location, symptom profile, and patient tolerance. Newer technologies, including directional leads and current steering, have expanded the ability to fine-tune stimulation fields, allowing clinicians to improve efficacy while reducing side effects such as dysarthria, paresthesias, or unwanted muscle contractions [53, 65].

Recognizing and managing stimulation-related side effects is a routine and important part of postoperative care. Motor effects may include dyskinesias, speech changes, or gait imbalance, while non-motor effects can involve mood shifts, anxiety, apathy, or cognitive fluctuations [45, 80]. Distinguishing stimulation effects from disease progression or medication changes requires careful longitudinal assessment and close communication among treating clinicians. Adjustments to stimulation parameters, medication regimens, or both are commonly needed to find the right balance.

Long-term success with DBS depends on sustained, multidisciplinary follow-up. Ongoing collaboration among movement disorder neurologists, functional neurosurgeons, and, when appropriate, psychiatrists and neuropsychologists is essential. Anesthesiologists may also remain involved for device-related procedures, generator replacements, or management of comorbid medical issues. Regular follow-up visits allow for timely programming adjustments, monitoring of disease progression, and early detection of hardware-related problems or emerging neuropsychiatric concerns [81]. In this way, DBS is best understood not as a one-time intervention but as a longitudinal therapy that evolves alongside the patient's disease.

8. Complications and risk mitigation

Even though DBS is a well-established and effective therapy, it carries a range of potential complications that span procedure- and hardware-related events, stimulation/programming effects, perioperative medical and anesthetic complications, and longer-term device issues. Understanding these risks and how they can be mitigated is central to patient safety and durable clinical benefit. Many complications are not attributable to a single factor but instead arise from the interaction between patient characteristics, disease severity, procedural technique, and perioperative management.

Surgical and hardware-related complications remain some of the most immediate concerns after DBS implantation. Intracranial hemorrhage, while uncommon, is among the most serious risks and is most often associated with lead placement or MER trajectories [71, 82]. Other complications include infection, lead migration, hardware malfunction, and skin erosion, which can present early or months after surgery [75, 76]. Hardware infections often require prolonged antibiotic therapy and may necessitate partial or complete system explantation. Risk reduction begins preoperatively with optimization of modifiable factors such as glycemic control, smoking cessation when feasible, and treatment of active skin infections. This is followed by standardized perioperative antibiotic prophylaxis timed to incision and redosed as appropriate for longer cases. Intraoperatively, meticulous sterile technique during tunneling and generator pocket creation, minimizing traffic and breaks in sterility, and careful hemostasis to prevent pocket hematomas are all important. After surgery, patient education on incision care and early evaluation of erythema, drainage, wound separation, or persistent pocket pain allows for timely intervention and may reduce progression to deep hardware infection. While advances in surgical technique and device design have lowered complication rates over time, ongoing vigilance remains key.

Neurologic and neuropsychiatric complications may result from both the surgical intervention and the effects of stimulation itself. Transient neurologic deficits can occur due to perioperative edema or microlesion effects, while stimulation-related symptoms may include dysarthria, paresthesias, gait imbalance, or visual disturbances [45, 80]. Neuropsychiatric effects like mood changes, anxiety, apathy, impulse control disorders, or cognitive decline are particularly relevant in susceptible patients and may be influenced by target choice, stimulation parameters, or preexisting psychiatric disease [34, 35, 83]. Careful preoperative screening, thoughtful target selection, and gradual, iterative postoperative programming are key strategies for reducing these risks.

Anesthesia-related complications represent another, sometimes underrecognized, source of morbidity in DBS surgery. Autonomic dysfunction is common in PD and increases the risk of perioperative hypotension, hypertension, and arrhythmias [52]. Sedatives and anesthetic agents can interfere with neurophysiologic monitoring, worsen motor symptoms, or contribute to postoperative confusion and delirium if not carefully chosen and titrated [51, 66]. Risk mitigation relies on anticipatory anesthetic planning, close communication with the surgical team, and avoidance of medications known to exacerbate parkinsonian symptoms or interact negatively with dopaminergic therapy [72].

Perioperative factors also shape long-term outcomes after DBS. Suboptimal lead placement, delayed or inconsistent programming, prolonged interruption of antiparkinsonian medications, and postoperative delirium have all been associated with reduced functional benefit and increased morbidity [73, 74, 84]. In contrast, coordinated perioperative care – marked by early mobilization, prompt medication resumption, and structured follow-up – meaningfully improves recovery and the durability of DBS benefits.

A practical framework for risk mitigation pairs common complications with early recognition cues and clear first-line responses. New focal neurologic deficits, severe headache, repeated vomiting, or unexplained delayed awakening should prompt urgent evaluation for intracranial hemorrhage and expedited neuroimaging. Fever, wound drainage, progressive erythema, or increasing pocket tenderness should raise concern for infection and trigger early surgical and infectious disease consultation. Prominent postoperative confusion, hallucinations, or agitation should lead to assessment for missed medications, metabolic abnormalities, sleep disruption, or pain, with management favoring nonpharmacologic delirium strategies and avoidance of dopamine-blocking agents. Hemodynamic instability may reflect underlying dysautonomia, and treatment focuses on careful titration of fluids and vasoactive medications to maintain cerebral perfusion while avoiding hypertension during periods of hemorrhage risk.

Taken together, complications associated with DBS are best viewed as part of a broader perioperative continuum rather than as isolated events. Effective risk reduction depends on careful patient selection, precise surgical technique, thoughtful anesthetic management, and sustained multidisciplinary follow-up. When these elements are aligned, the risks of DBS can be substantially reduced, allowing patients to achieve the greatest and most durable benefit from this advanced therapy.

9. Emerging innovations and future directions

DBS for PD is continuing to move beyond traditional open-loop approaches, driven forward by advances in neural sensing, imaging, and device technology. Conventional DBS delivers continuous stimulation using fixed parameters, but newer strategies focus on improving precision, limiting side effects, and better matching stimulation to the underlying disease biology. These changes reflect a broader shift toward more personalized, circuit-based neuromodulation.

One of the most notable developments is the rise of adaptive, or closed-loop, DBS systems. Adaptive DBS uses real-time neural signals – most commonly beta-band local field potentials, particularly in STN DBS – as control inputs to adjust stimulation dynamically in response to pathologic brain activity [59, 85, 86]. Instead of stimulating continuously, these systems target periods of abnormal synchronization. Alternative biomarkers and multi-signal approaches are also being explored, reflecting clinical heterogeneity across patients, phenotypes, and targets. Early work suggests this approach can improve motor control while reducing stimulation-related side effects and overall energy use [39]. Initial clinical studies and proof-of-concept trials have shown promising results, particularly for managing motor fluctuations, though larger and longer-term studies are still needed.

Advances in imaging and connectomic targeting are also changing how DBS is planned and how outcomes are understood. High-resolution structural MRI, diffusion tractography, and network-level analyses now make it possible to visualize patient-specific connectivity within basal ganglia–thalamocortical circuits [52, 87]. Rather than focusing on individual nuclei alone, newer approaches increasingly emphasize modulation of functional networks tied to symptom expression. Connectomic analyses have been linked to clinical outcomes, offering a way to refine both target selection and postoperative programming in a more systematic way [39, 88].

Hardware innovations in neuromodulation have further expanded what DBS can do. Directional leads allow current steering, giving clinicians more control over stimulation fields and helping avoid nearby structures associated with adverse effects [53, 65]. Devices capable of chronic neural sensing provide ongoing physiologic data, which can inform programming decisions over time and support adaptive stimulation algorithms [59, 89]. As these technologies mature, the line between neuromodulation and brain–computer interface concepts is starting to blur, opening the door to more individualized therapy.

Perioperative and anesthetic care will also need to evolve alongside these advances. As neural sensing and adaptive stimulation become more central to DBS systems, anesthetic strategies must consider how sedatives, anesthetic agents, physiologic variables, and perioperative medication management influence recorded neural signals and network behavior [51, 66]. Standardizing these conditions – especially during recording-driven implantation, biomarker calibration, or early programming – may help improve signal quality and closed-loop performance. Closer collaboration among anesthesiologists, neurologists, neurosurgeons, and biomedical engineers will be increasingly important to ensure that perioperative management supports both surgical accuracy and the performance of emerging closed-loop technologies.

Collectively, these developments point toward a shift away from static stimulation and toward dynamic, circuit-informed neuromodulation. Continued integration of adaptive systems, advanced imaging, and coordinated multidisciplinary care has the potential to further improve outcomes and broaden the therapeutic reach of DBS for patients with PD.

10. Conclusion

DBS has become a core therapeutic option for patients with PD whose motor symptoms are no longer well-controlled with medication alone. By directly modulating dysfunctional basal ganglia–thalamocortical circuits, DBS provides sustained improvement in motor function, reduces medication-related complications, and meaningfully improves quality of life. Its effectiveness does not hinge on any single technical step; instead, it depends on how well neurobiologic insight, patient selection, surgical execution, anesthetic management, and long-term follow-up are brought together.

Throughout this chapter, DBS has been framed as a fundamentally multidisciplinary therapy. Advances in functional neurosurgery and device technology have widened what is possible, but those gains are only fully realized when surgical strategy is closely aligned with perioperative anesthetic care. Anesthetic decisions shape intraoperative neurophysiology and perioperative conditions that support accurate targeting, patient safety, and postoperative recovery. For that reason, anesthetic care is more than logistical support in DBS surgery – it is an integral component of the overall DBS workflow. Close collaboration among anesthesiologists, neurologists, and neurosurgeons is essential to achieving the best outcomes.

From a clinical standpoint, integrating surgical and anesthetic approaches helps create the conditions for accurate lead placement, effective programming, and safe recovery. Choices around target selection, procedural technique, intraoperative physiologic management, and postoperative programming interact and can influence both therapeutic benefit and side-effect burden. Viewing DBS as a dynamic, longitudinal therapy underscores the importance of structured follow-up, iterative programming, and ongoing reassessment as PD progresses.

Looking ahead, continued advances in adaptive stimulation, imaging-guided targeting, and neuromodulation hardware are likely to further refine DBS as a personalized, circuit-informed therapy. These developments will place even greater emphasis on multidisciplinary expertise and coordinated perioperative care. As functional neurosurgery and anesthetic practice continue to evolve alongside emerging technologies, DBS will remain a cornerstone of advanced PD management and a clear example of what integrated, patient-centered care can achieve.

Acknowledgments

The authors acknowledge the use of OpenAI's ChatGPT 5.2 for language polishing of the manuscript.

Conflict of Interest

The authors declare no conflict of interest.

Author details

Nicholas Sookhoo[1], Ivy Zhou[2] and Jie Zhou[2*]

1 SUNY Downstate Medical Center, Brooklyn, USA

2 Brigham and Women's Hospital, Mass General Brigham, Boston, USA

*Address all correspondence to: jzhou@mgh.harvard.edu

References

[1] Kalia LV, Lang AE. Parkinson's disease. The Lancet. 2015;**386** (9996):896–912. DOI: 10.1016/S0140-6736(14)61393-3

[2] Olanow CW, Stern MB, Sethi K. The scientific and clinical basis for the treatment of Parkinson disease. Neurology. 2009;**72**(21 Suppl 4): S1–S136. DOI: 10.1212/WNL.0b013e3181a1d44c

[3] Obeso JA, Olanow CW, Nutt JG. Levodopa motor complications in Parkinson's disease. Trends in Neurosciences. 2000;**23**(10 Suppl):S2–S7. DOI: 10.1016/S0166-2236(00)01643-9

[4] Poewe W, Seppi K, Tanner CM, et al. Parkinson disease. Nature Reviews Disease Primers. 2017;**3**:17013. DOI: 10.1038/nrdp.2017.13

[5] Benabid AL, Pollak P, Gross C, et al. Acute and long-term effects of subthalamic nucleus stimulation in Parkinson's disease. The Lancet 1994;**343**:91–95. DOI: 10.1016/S0140-6736(94)90944-8

[6] Deuschl G, Schade-Brittinger C, Krack P, et al. A randomized trial of deep-brain stimulation for Parkinson's disease. New England Journal of Medicine. 2006;**355**:896–908. DOI: 10.1056/NEJMoa060281

[7] Weaver FM, Follett K, Stern M, et al. Bilateral deep brain stimulation vs best medical therapy for patients with advanced Parkinson disease. Jama. 2009;**301**:63–73. DOI: 10.1001/jama.2008.929.

[8] Okun MS. Deep-brain stimulation for Parkinson's disease. New England Journal of Medicine. 2012;**367**(16):1529–1538. DOI: 10.1056/NEJMct1208070

[9] Bronstein JM, Tagliati M, Alterman RL, et al. Deep brain stimulation for Parkinson disease: An expert consensus. Archives of Neurology. 2011;**68**:165–171. DOI: 10.1001/archneurol.2010.260

[10] Venkatraghavan L, Luciano M, Manninen P. Anesthetic management of patients undergoing deep brain stimulator insertion. Anesthesia & Analgesia. 2010;**110**(4):1138–1145. DOI: 10.1213/ANE.0b013e3181cc5f85

[11] Fluchère F, Witjas T, Eusebio A, et al. Controlled general anaesthesia for subthalamic nucleus stimulation in Parkinson's disease. Journal of Neurology, Neurosurgery & Psychiatry. 2014;**85**:1162–1168. DOI: 10.1136/jnnp-2013-305323

[12] Albin RL, Young AB, Penney JB. The functional anatomy of basal ganglia disorders. Trends in Neurosciences. 1989;**12**(10):366–375. DOI: 10.1016/0166-2236(89)90074-X

[13] DeLong MR, Wichmann T. Circuits and circuit disorders of the basal ganglia. Archives of Neurology. 2007;**64** (1):20–24. DOI: 10.1001/archneur.64.1.20

[14] Obeso JA, Rodriguez-Oroz MC, Benitez-Temino B, et al. Functional organization of the basal ganglia. Movement Disorders 2008;**23**:S548–S559. DOI: 10.1002/mds.22077

[15] Alexander GE, DeLong MR, Strick PL. Parallel organization of functionally segregated circuits linking basal ganglia and cortex. Annual Review of

Neuroscience. 1986;**9**:357–381. DOI: 10.1146/annurev.ne.09.030186.002041

[16] Gerfen CR, Surmeier DJ. Modulation of striatal projection systems by dopamine. Annual Review of Neuroscience. 2011;**34**:441–466. DOI: 10.1146/annurev-neuro-061010-113641

[17] DeLong MR. Primate models of movement disorders of basal ganglia origin. Trends in Neurosciences. 1990;**13**(7):281–285. DOI: 10.1016/0166-2236(90)90110-V

[18] Brown P. Abnormal oscillatory synchronisation in the motor system. Current Opinion in Neurobiology. 2007;**17**(6):656–664. DOI: 10.1016/j.conb.2007.12.001

[19] Hammond C, Bergman H, Brown P. Pathological synchronization in Parkinson's disease. Trends in Neurosciences. 2007;**30**(7):357–364. DOI: 10.1016/j.tins.2007.05.004

[20] Little S, Brown P. The functional role of beta oscillations in Parkinson's disease. Parkinsonism & Related Disorders. 2014;**20**(Suppl 1):S44–S48. DOI: 10.1016/S1353-8020(13)70013-0

[21] Kühn AA, Kupsch A, Schneider GH, Brown P. Reduction in subthalamic 8-35 Hz oscillatory activity correlates with clinical improvement in Parkinson's disease. The European Journal of Neuroscience. 2006;**23**(7):1956–1960. DOI: 10.1111/j.1460-9568.2006.04717.x

[22] Vitek JL. Mechanisms of deep brain stimulation. Movement Disorders. 2002;**17**(S3):S69–S72. DOI: 10.1002/mds.10144

[23] McIntyre CC, Savasta M, Kerkerian-Le Goff L, Vitek JL. Uncovering the mechanism(s) of action of deep brain stimulation: Activation, inhibition, or both. Clinical Neurophysiology. 2004;**115**(6):1239–1248. DOI: 10.1016/j.clinph.2003.12.024

[24] Eusebio A, Brown P. Synchronisation in the beta frequency-band — The bad boy of parkinsonism or an innocent bystander. Experimental Neurology. 2009;**217**(1):1–3. DOI: 10.1016/j.expneurol.2009.02.003

[25] Larson PS. Deep brain stimulation for movement disorders. Neurotherapeutics. 2014;**11**(3):465–474. DOI: 10.1007/s13311-014-0274-1

[26] Charles PD, Padaliya BB, Newman WJ, Gill CE, Covington CD, Fang JY, So SA, Tramontana MG, Konrad PE, Davis TL. Deep brain stimulation of the subthalamic nucleus reduces antiparkinsonian medication costs. Parkinsonism and Related Disorders. 2004;**10**(8):475–479. DOI: 10.1016/j.parkreldis.2004.05.006

[27] Limousin P, Foltynie T. Long-term outcomes of deep brain stimulation in Parkinson disease. Nature Reviews Neurology. 2019;**15**(4):234–242. DOI: 10.1038/s41582-019-0145-9

[28] Schuepbach WMM, Rau J, Knudsen K, et al; EARLYSTIM Study Group. Neurostimulation for Parkinson's disease with early motor complications. The New England Journal of Medicine (NEJM). 2013;**368**(7):610–622. DOI: 10.1056/NEJMoa1205158

[29] Fasano A, Herzog J, Seifert E, Stolze H, Falk D, Reese R, Volkmann J, Deuschl G. Modulation of gait coordination by subthalamic stimulation improves freezing of gait. Movement Disorders. 2011;**26**(5):844–851. DOI: 10.1002/mds.23583

[30] Witt K, Daniels C, Reiff J, et al. Neuropsychological and psychiatric changes after deep brain stimulation for Parkinson's disease: A randomised, multicentre study. Lancet Neurology. 2008;**7**(7):605–614. DOI: 10.1016/S147 4-4422(08)70114-5

[31] Zheng Y, Wei L, Ang SYL, Ng HL, Au WL, Tay KY, Xu Z, Ng WH, Tan LCS, Neo SX, Wan KR. Outcomes after deep brain stimulation for elderly versus non-elderly patients with Parkinson's disease. Clinical Neurology and Neurosurgery. 2024;**242**:108319. DOI: 1 0.1016/j.clineuro.2024.108319

[32] Williams DR, Litvan I. Parkinsonian syndromes. Continuum. 2013;**19**(5):1189–1212. DOI: 10.1212/01. CON.0000436152.24038.e0

[33] Accolla EA, Pollo C. Mood effects after deep brain stimulation for Parkinson's disease: an update. Front Neurol. 2019;**10**:617. DOI: 10.3389/ fneur.2019.00617

[34] Parsons TD, Rogers SA, Braaten AJ, Woods SP, Tröster AI. Cognitive sequelae of subthalamic nucleus deep brain stimulation in Parkinson's disease: a meta-analysis. Lancet Neurology. 2006;**5**(7):578–588. DOI: 10.1016/ S1474-4422(06)70475-6

[35] Smeding HMM, Speelman JD, Koning-Haanstra M, Schuurman PR, Nijssen P, van Laar T, Schmand B. Neuropsychological effects of bilateral STN stimulation in Parkinson disease: A controlled study. Neurology. 2006;**66** (12):1830–1836. DOI: 10.1212/01. wnl.0000234881.77830.66

[36] Starr PA, Christine CW, Theodosopoulos PV, Lindsey N, Byrd D, Moseley A, Marks WJ Jr. Implantation of deep brain stimulators into the subthalamic nucleus: technical approach and magnetic resonance imaging-verified lead locations. Journal of neurosurgery. 2002;**97**(2):370–387. DOI: 10.3171/jns.2002.97.2.0370

[37] Krack P, Batir A, Van Blercom N, Chabardes S, Fraix V, Ardouin C, Koudsie A, Dowsey-Limousin P, Benazzouz A, LeBas JF, Benabid AL, Pollak P. Five-year follow-up of bilateral stimulation of the subthalamic nucleus in advanced Parkinson's disease. The New England Journal of Medicine (NEJM). 2003;**349**(20):1925–1934. DOI: 10.1056/NEJMoa035275

[38] Anderson VC, Burchiel KJ, Hogarth P, Favre J, Hammerstad JP. Pallidal vs subthalamic nucleus deep brain stimulation in Parkinson disease. Archives of Neurology. 2005;**62**(4):554–560. DOI: 10.1001/archneur.62.4.554

[39] Horn A, Reich M, Vorwerk J, et al. Connectivity Predicts deep brain stimulation outcome in Parkinson disease. Annals of Neurology 2017;**82**:67–78. DOI: 10.1002/ana.24974

[40] Temel Y, Kessels A, Tan S, Topdag A, Boon P, Visser-Vandewalle V. Behavioural changes after bilateral subthalamic stimulation in advanced Parkinson disease: A systematic review. Parkinsonism and Related Disorders. 2006;**12**(5):265–272. DOI: 10.1016/j. parkreldis.2006.01.004

[41] Odekerken VJJ, Boel JA, Schmand BA, de Haan RJ, Figee M, van den Munckhof P, Schuurman PR, de Bie RMA; NSTAPS Study Group. GPi vs STN deep brain stimulation for Parkinson disease: Three-year follow-up. Neurology. 2016;**86**(8):755–761. DOI: 10. 1212/WNL.0000000000002401

[42] Follett KA, Weaver FM, Stern M, Hur K, Harris CL, Luo P, Marks WJ Jr, Rothlind J, Sagher O, Moy C, Pahwa R, Burchiel K, Hogarth P, Lai EC, Duda JE, Holloway K, Samii A, Horn S, Bronstein JM, Stoner G, Starr PA, Simpson R, Baltuch G, De Salles A, Huang GD, Reda DJ; CSP 468 Study Group. Pallidal versus subthalamic deep-brain stimulation for Parkinson's disease. The New England Journal of Medicine. 2010;**362**(22):2077–2091. DOI: 10.1056/NEJMoa0907083

[43] Benabid AL, Pollak P, Gervason C, Hoffmann D, Gao DM, Hommel M, Perret JE, de Rougemont J. Long-term suppression of tremor by chronic stimulation of the ventral intermediate thalamic nucleus. Lancet. 1991;**337**(8738):403–406. DOI: 10.1016/0140-6736(91)91175-T

[44] Moro E, Hamani C, Poon YY, Al-Khairallah T, Dostrovsky JO, Hutchison WD, Lozano AM. Unilateral pedunculopontine stimulation improves falls in Parkinson's disease. Brain. 2010;**133**(Pt 1):215–224. DOI: 10.1093/brain/awp261

[45] Abosch A, Timmermann L, Bartley S, Rietkerk HG, Whiting D, Connolly PJ, Lanctin D, Hariz MI. An international survey of deep brain stimulation procedural steps. Stereotactic Functional Neurosurgery. 2013;**91**(1):1–11. DOI: 10.1159/000343207

[46] Zrinzo L, Foltynie T, Limousin P, Hariz MI. Reducing hemorrhagic complications. Journal of Neurosurgery. 2012;**116**(1):84–94. DOI: 10.3171/2011.8.JNS101407

[47] Raz A, Eimerl D, Zaidel A, Bergman H, Israel Z. Propofol decreases neuronal population spiking activity in the subthalamic nucleus of Parkinsonian patients. Anesthesia and Analgesia. 2010;**111**(5):1285–1289. DOI: 10.1213/ANE.0b013e3181f565f2

[48] Bekker AY, Kaufman B, Samir H, Doyle W. The use of dexmedetomidine infusion for awake craniotomy. Anesthesia and Analgesia. 2001;**92**(5):1251–1253. DOI: 10.1097/00000539-200105000-00031

[49] Elias WJ, Durieux ME, Huss D, Frysinger RC. Dexmedetomidine and arousal affect subthalamic neurons. Movement Disorders. 2008;**23**(9): 1317–1320. DOI: 10.1002/mds.22080.

[50] Murselović T, Makovšek A. Airway management in neuroanesthesia. Acta Clinica Croatica. 2023;**62**(Suppl 1):119–124. DOI: 10.20471/acc.2023.62.s1.15

[51] Goldstein DS. Dysautonomia in Parkinson disease. Comprehensive Physiology. 2014;**4**(2):805–826. DOI: 10.1002/cphy.c130026.

[52] Newman EJ, Grosset DG, Kennedy PGE. The parkinsonism-hyperpyrexia syndrome. Neurocritical care. 2009;**10**(1):136–140. DOI: 10.1007/s12028-008-9125-4

[53] Li H, Han S, Feng J. Delirium after deep brain stimulation in Parkinson's disease. Parkinson's disease. 2021;**2021**: 8885386. DOI: 10.1155/2021/8885386

[54] Castrioto A, Lozano AM, Poon YY, Lang AE, Fallis M, Moro E. Ten-year outcome of subthalamic stimulation in Parkinson disease: A blinded evaluation. Archives of Neurology. 2011;**68**(12):1550–1556. DOI: 10.1001/archneurol.2011.182

[55] Little S, Brown P. What brain signals are suitable for feedback control of deep brain stimulation in Parkinson's disease? Annals of the New

York Academy of Sciences. 2012;**1265** (1):9–24. DOI: 10.1111/j. 1749-6632.2012.06650.x

[56] Swann NC, de Hemptinne C, Miocinovic S, Qasim S, Ostrem JL, Galifianakis NB, San Luciano M, Wang SS, Ziman N, Taylor R, Starr PA. Chronic multisite brain recordings from a totally implantable bidirectional neural interface: experience in 5 patients with Parkinson's disease. Journal of Neurosurgery. 2018;**128**(2):605–616. DOI: 10.3171/2016.11.JNS161162

[57] Rosin B, Slovik M, Mitelman R, Rivlin-Etzion M, Haber SN, Israel Z, Vaadia E, Bergman H. Closed-loop deep brain stimulation is superior in ameliorating parkinsonism. Neuron. 2011;**72**(2):370–384. DOI: 10.1016/j. neuron.2011.08.023

[58] Arlotti M, Marceglia S, Foffani G, Volkmann J, Lozano AM, Moro E, Cogiamanian F, Prenassi M, Bocci T, Cortese F, Rampini P, Barbieri S, Priori A. Eight-hours adaptive deep brain stimulation in patients with Parkinson disease. Neurology. 2018;**90**(11): e971–e976. DOI: 10.1212/ WNL.0000000000005121

[59] Neumann WJ, Turner RS, Blankertz B, Mitchell T, Kühn AA, Richardson RM. Toward electrophysiology-based intelligent adaptive deep brain stimulation for movement disorders. Neurotherapeutics. 2019;**16**(1):105–118. DOI: 10.1007/s13311-018-00705-0

[60] Chen T, Mirzadeh Z, Chapple KM, Lambert M, Shill HA, Moguel-Cobos G, Tröster AI, Dhall R, Ponce FA. Clinical outcomes following awake and asleep deep brain stimulation for Parkinson disease. Journal of Neurosurgery. 2018;**130**(1):109–120. DOI: 10.3171/201 7.8.JNS17883

[61] Brodsky MA, Anderson S, Murchison C, Seier M, Wilhelm J, Vederman A, Burchiel KJ. Clinical outcomes of asleep vs awake deep brain stimulation for Parkinson disease. Neurology. 2017;**89**(19):1944–1950. DOI: 10.1212/WNL.00000000 00004630

[62] Bos MJ, Buhre W, Temel Y, Joosten EAJ, Absalom AR, Janssen MLF. Effect of anesthesia on microelectrode recordings during deep brain stimulation surgery: A narrative review. Journal of Neurosurgical Anesthesiology. 2021;**33**(4):300–307. DOI: 10.1097/ANA.00000000 00000673

[63] Maltête D, Jodoin N, Karachi C, Houeto JL, Navarro S, Cornu P, Agid Y, Welter ML. Subthalamic stimulation and neuronal activity in the substantia nigra in Parkinson's disease. Journal of Neurophysiology. 2007;**97**(6):4017–4022. DOI: 10.1152/ jn.01104.2006

[64] Cho ZH, Min HK, Oh SH, Han JY, Park CW, Chi JG, Kim YB, Paek SH, Lozano AM, Lee KH. Direct visualization of deep brain stimulation targets using MRI. Neuroimage. 2010;**54** (3):1909–1918. DOI: 10.1016/j. neuroimage.2010.09.014

[65] Steigerwald F, Müller L, Johannes S, Matthies C, Volkmann J. Directional deep brain stimulation of the subthalamic nucleus: A pilot study using a novel neurostimulation device. Movement Disorders. 2016;**31**(8): 1240–1243. DOI: 10.1002/mds.26669

[66] Raz A, Eimerl D, Zaidel A, Bergman H, Israel Z. Propofol decreases

neuronal population spiking activity in the subthalamic nucleus of Parkinsonian patients. Anesthesia and Analgesia. 2010;**111**(5):1285–1289. DOI: 10.1213/ANE.0b013e3181f565f2

[67] Prontera A, Baroni S, Marudi A, Valzania F, Feletti A, Benuzzi F, Bertellini E, Pavesi G. Awake craniotomy anesthetic management using dexmedetomidine, propofol, and remifentanil. Drug Design, Development and Therap. 2017;**11**:593–598. DOI: 10.2147/DDDT.S124736

[68] Bekker AY, Kaufman B, Samir H, Doyle W. The use of dexmedetomidine infusion for awake craniotomy. Anesth Analg. 2001;**92**(5):1251–1253. DOI: 10.1097/00000539-200105000-00031

[69] Bekker AY, Kaufman B, Samir H, Doyle W. The use of dexmedetomidine infusion for awake craniotomy. Anesthesia and Analgesia. 2001;**92**(5):1251–1253. DOI: 10.1097/00000539-200105000-00031

[70] Zrinzo L, Foltynie T, Limousin P, Hariz MI. Reducing hemorrhagic complications in functional neurosurgery: a large case series and systematic literature review. Journal of Neurosurgery. 2012;**116**(1):84–94. DOI: 10.3171/2011.8.JNS101407.

[71] Hu SC, Frucht SJ. Emergency treatment of movement disorders. Curr Treat Options Neurol. 2007;**9**(2):103–114. DOI: 10.1007/s11940-007-0036-z

[72] Carlson JD, Neumiller JJ, Swain LDW, Mark J, McLeod P, Hirschauer J. Postoperative delirium in Parkinson's disease patients following deep brain stimulation surgery. Journal of Clinical Neuroscience. 2014;**21**(7):1192–1195. DOI: 10.1016/j.jocn.2013.12.007

[73] Fenoy AJ, Simpson RK Jr. Risks of common complications in deep brain stimulation surgery: management and avoidance. Journal of Neurosurgery. 2014;**120**(1):132–139. DOI: 10.3171/2013.10.JNS131225

[74] Voges J, Waerzeggers Y, Maarouf M, Lehrke R, Koulousakis A, Lenartz D, Sturm V. Deep-brain stimulation: long-term analysis of complications caused by hardware and surgery—experiences from a single centre. Journal of Neurology, Neurosurgery and Psychiatry. 2006;**77**(7):868–872. DOI: 10.1136/jnnp.2005.081232

[75] Binder DK, Rau GM, Starr PA. Risk factors for hemorrhage during microelectrode-guided deep brain stimulator implantation for movement disorders. Neurosurgery. 2005;**56**(4):722–732. DOI: 10.1227/01.NEU.0000156473.57196.7E

[76] Appleby BS, Duggan PS, Regenberg A, Rabins PV. Psychiatric and neuropsychiatric adverse events associated with deep brain stimulation: a meta-analysis of ten years' experience. Movement Disorders. 2007;**22**(12):1722–1728. DOI: 10.1002/mds.21551.

[77] Castrioto A, Lozano AM, Poon YY, Lang AE, Fallis M, Moro E. Ten-year outcome of subthalamic stimulation in Parkinson disease: A blinded evaluation. Archives of Neurology. 2011;**68**(12):1550–1556. DOI: 10.1001/archneurol.2011.182.

[78] Moro E, Esselink RJA, Xie J, Hommel M, Benabid AL, Pollak P. The impact on Parkinson's disease of electrical parameter settings in STN stimulation. Neurology. 2002;**59**(5):706–713. DOI: 10.1212/WNL.59.5.706.

[79] Volkmann J, Moro E, Pahwa R. Basic algorithms for the programming of deep brain stimulation in Parkinson's disease. Movement Disorders. 2006;**21** (Suppl 14):S284–S289. DOI: 10.1002/mds.20961

[80] McIntyre CC, Foutz TJ. Computational modeling of deep brain stimulation. Handbook of Clinical Neurology. 2013;**116**:55–61. DOI: 10.1016/B978-0-444-53497-2.00005-X

[81] Hariz MI, Rehncrona S, Quinn NP, Speelman JD, Wensing C; Multicentre Advanced Parkinson's Disease Deep Brain Stimulation Group. Multicenter study on deep brain stimulation in Parkinson's disease: An independent assessment of reported adverse events at 4 years. Movement Disorders. 2008;**23** (3):416–421. DOI: 10.1002/mds.21888

[82] Little S, Brown P. What brain signals are suitable for feedback control of deep brain stimulation in Parkinson's disease? Annals of the New York Academy of Sciences. 2012;**1265** (1):9–24. DOI: 10.1111/j.1749-6632.2012.06650.x

[83] Stanslaski SR, Case MA, Giftakis JE, Raike RS, Stypulkowski PH. Long term performance of a bi-directional neural interface for deep brain stimulation and recording. Frontiers in Human Neuroscience. 2022;**16**:916627. DOI: 10.3389/fnhum.2022.916627

[84] Rosin B, Slovik M, Mitelman R, Rivlin-Etzion M, Haber SN, Israel Z, Vaadia E, Bergman H. Closed-loop deep brain stimulation is superior in ameliorating parkinsonism. Neuron. 2011;**72**(2):370–384. DOI: 10.1016/j.neuron.2011.08.023

[85] Arlotti M, Marceglia S, Foffani G, Volkmann J, Lozano AM, Moro E, Cogiamanian F, Prenassi M, Bocci T, Cortese F, Rampini P, Barbieri S, Priori A. Eight-hours adaptive deep brain stimulation in patients with Parkinson disease. Neurology. 2018;**90**(11):e971–e976. DOI: 10.1212/WNL.0000000000005121

[86] Coenen VA, Schlaepfer TE, Allert N, et al. Diffusion tensor imaging and neuromodulation: DTI as key technology for deep brain stimulation. 2015;**38**:E10. DOI: 10.1016/B978-0-12-404706-8.00011-5

[87] Pollo C, Kaelin-Lang A, Oertel MF, Stieglitz L, Taub E, Fuhr P, Lozano AM, Raabe A, Schüpbach M. Directional deep brain stimulation: An intraoperative double-blind pilot study. Brain. 2014;**137**(Pt 7):2015–2026. DOI: 10.1093/brain/awu102

[88] Steigerwald F, Matthies C, Volkmann J. Directional deep brain stimulation of the subthalamic nucleus: A pilot study using a novel neurostimulation device. Movement Disorders: Official Journal of the Movement Disorder Society. 2019;**34** (11):1585–1595. DOI: 10.1002/mds.26669

[89] Horn A, Neumann WJ. From adaptive deep brain stimulation to adaptive circuit targeting. Nature Reviews Neurology. 2025;**21** (10):556–566. DOI: 10.1038/s41582-025-01131-5

Chapter 5

Advanced Deep Brain Stimulation Strategies for Cervical Dystonia and Dystonic Tremor in the Context of Parkinson's Disease: Current Perspectives and Future Directions

Akın Akakın, Emre Ünal and Abdullah Andaç

Abstract

Cervical dystonia and dystonic tremor are two complex motor symptoms of Parkinson's disease (PD) that can challenge its diagnosis and treatment. Recent studies suggest their pathophysiology as a network disorder involving the basal ganglia, cerebellum, thalamus, and cortex, rather than a pure dopaminergic deficit. Despite the potential benefits of standard therapeutic modalities such as dopaminergic optimization, botulinum toxin, and rehabilitation, some patients continue to experience significant disability. Deep brain stimulation (DBS) is a significant therapeutic alternative in such cases. The target of the stimulation is selected according to the main clinical problem: GPi for dystonia, VIM for tremor, and STN for the motor symptoms of PD. Recent advances focus on adaptive DBS, directional leads, connectomic targeting, and AI-assisted programming, enabling more individualized neuromodulation. This chapter reviews the pathophysiology, clinical features, and advanced DBS approaches for cervical dystonia and dystonic tremor in PD.

Keywords: deep brain stimulation, Parkinson's disease, cervical dystonia, dystonic tremor, basal ganglia

1. Introduction

Parkinson's disease (PD) is a progressive neurodegenerative disorder characterized by classical motor symptoms, including resting tremor, bradykinesia, and rigidity [1]. However, the clinical spectrum of PD extends beyond these major features, encompassing a diverse set of motor and non-motor manifestations that significantly contribute to reduced quality of life and disability. Among these, cervical dystonia and dystonic tremor represent particularly challenging and often underrecognized motor phenotypes that can complicate diagnostic assessment and therapeutic decision-making in PD patients [2, 3].

Cervical dystonia is characterized by involuntary, sustained or intermittent contractions of the neck muscles, leading to abnormal head postures and movements. In PD, it may present as an "off"-period phenomenon, a peak-dose complication, or a persistent motor feature that is unresponsive to optimized dopaminergic therapy [4]. Dystonic tremor is defined as tremor occurring in body regions with dystonia. It is frequently seen in PD and can be challenging to distinguish from essential tremor or parkinsonian rest tremor, as it often exhibits distinct characteristics such as asymmetry and irregularity [5]. These clinical features highlight the limitations of conventional pharmacological approaches and emphasize the need for advanced therapeutic interventions [6]. Deep Brain Stimulation (DBS) is an established and remarkably effective neurosurgical treatment for numerous conditions, including essential tremor and primary dystonia [7]. Over the past two decades, DBS has evolved from a nucleus-centered approach to a broader network-based understanding of neuromodulation. This shift reflects the recognition that movement disorders arise from dysfunction within distributed neural circuits involving the basal ganglia, cerebellum, and cortical regions, rather than from isolated structures [8].

Modern DBS was first introduced in the late 1980s, and subsequent advancements in hardware, software, imaging, and physiological understanding have expanded its clinical use and improved its effectiveness [7, 9]. Recent breakthroughs, including adaptive DBS (aDBS) and connectomic targeting, are paving the way for personalized neuromodulation strategies tailored to individual patient neurophysiology and clinical presentation [10]. These innovations hold immense promise for optimizing outcomes in complex movement disorders.

This chapter reviews advanced DBS strategies for the management of cervical dystonia and dystonic tremor in PD, with a focus on pathophysiology, patient selection, target identification, and programming approaches. It also highlights the growing role of personalized neuromodulation, adaptive DBS, and emerging technologies, while addressing current challenges and future directions in this evolving field. By integrating mechanistic insights with clinical considerations, this chapter aims to provide a practical framework to improve therapeutic outcomes.

2. Pathophysiology of cervical dystonia and dystonic tremor in PD

The pathophysiology of cervical dystonia and dystonic tremor within the spectrum of PD is increasingly understood through a network-centric rather than a purely nucleus-centric model. These complex motor phenotypes are not merely a direct consequence of dopamine deficiency in the basal ganglia but rather stem from widespread dysfunction within interconnected cortico-basal ganglia-cerebellar circuits. This evolving understanding highlights the intricate interplay between various brain regions that contribute to the manifestation of these challenging symptoms [11].

2.1 Basal ganglia dysfunction

The hallmark of PD is the degeneration of dopaminergic neurons in the substantia nigra pars compacta, leading to a notable reduction in dopamine levels in the striatum. This reduction causes the disruption of the intricate balance of the basal ganglia's direct and indirect pathways, which is traditionally associated with core PD motor symptoms such as bradykinesia and rigidity [11]. However, aberrant basal ganglia activity also plays a critical role in the pathophysiology of dystonia [12].

Dystonia in PD is thought to be a consequence of the loss of inhibition pathways within the basal ganglia, particularly in the globus pallidus. This leads to excessive and uncoordinated output from the basal ganglia to the thalamus and subsequently to the motor cortex. Abnormal firing patterns, often characterized by bursts and pauses, contribute to the sustained muscle contractions and overflow phenomena characteristic of dystonia. Specific patterns of dopamine dysregulation may selectively affect inhibitory circuits, leading to dystonic postures or movements. These can occur during "off" periods, when dopaminergic tone is low, or as peak-dose dyskinesias, when dopaminergic stimulation is excessive. Furthermore, impaired sensorimotor integration within the basal ganglia, crucial for combining sensory information with motor commands, can lead to abnormal internal models of movement and distorted body representations [13, 14]

2.2 Cerebellar involvement: The two-node network hypothesis

The role of the cerebellum was underestimated, with primary focus on the basal ganglia. Recent evidence suggests that cerebellar dysfunction, along with its connections to the basal ganglia and cortex, plays an important role in the pathogenesis of dystonia and dystonic tremor [11, 15].

The "two-node network hypothesis" emphasizes the pathological interaction between two major network hubs: the basal ganglia and the cerebellum, which causes dystonic tremor. In this model, dystonia-related abnormal pallidal output creates a permissive state for tremor generation, while cerebellar circuits act as the primary oscillatory driver of tremor via the dentato-rubro-thalamic tract. Functional imaging studies have demonstrated abnormal activation and connectivity within cerebellar and sensorimotor cortical regions in patients with dystonic tremor. Electrophysiological recordings show tremor-related oscillations that are more consistent with cerebellothalamic rather than pallidal activity, supporting the involvement of both networks [16]. Dysfunction within the cerebello-thalamo-cortical circuit and the pallidum involves both functional and structural changes, including reduced cerebellar input to thalamocortical pathways and possible thalamic hypertrophy [17].

2.3 Thalamic and cortical contributions

The thalamus serves as a critical relay station, integrating inputs from both the basal ganglia and cerebellum before projecting to the motor cortex. Abnormal oscillatory activity within specific thalamic nuclei, particularly the ventral intermediate nucleus (VIM), is closely associated with tremor generation. In dystonic tremor, abnormal input to the VIM from the cerebello-thalamo-cortical pathway contributes to tremor [18, 19].

At the cortical level, functional imaging studies in dystonia often reveal abnormal activation patterns in primary and supplementary motor cortices, prefrontal areas, and parietal regions. These alterations suggest impaired cortical inhibition, abnormal sensorimotor processing, and disrupted motor planning and execution. The co-occurrence of PD can further exacerbate these cortical dysfunctions due to widespread neurodegenerative changes and altered neuromodulatory influences. Moreover, specific cortical territories for parkinsonism and dystonia have been suggested, with parkinsonism originating in a secondary motor subcircuit and dystonia in a primary motor cortical-basal ganglia subcircuit [18, 19].

In summary, cervical dystonia and dystonic tremor in PD are manifestations of a broader network dysfunction, extending beyond isolated basal ganglia pathology to encompass complex interactions involving the cerebellum, thalamus, and cortex. This network-based understanding is fundamental for developing targeted neuromodulation strategies [19, 20].

3. Clinical phenotypes and diagnostic considerations

Accurate diagnosis and phenotyping of cervical dystonia and dystonic tremor in the context of PD are crucial for guiding therapeutic decisions, particularly when considering advanced neuromodulation strategies. The clinical presentation can be heterogeneous, and careful differentiation from other movement disorders and Parkinsonian symptoms is essential [21].

3.1 Cervical dystonia in PD

Cervical dystonia in PD can manifest in several ways, often complicating the motor profile of the disease. It typically presents as sustained or intermittent contractions of the neck muscles, leading to abnormal head movements or postures such as torticollis, retrocollis, laterocollis, or anterocollis. These manifestations can vary significantly in their relationship to dopaminergic therapy and disease progression [4].

- **"Off-Period" Dystonia:** This common manifestation occurs during periods of low dopaminergic medication levels. It is often painful, sustained, and posture-dominant, reflecting impaired basal ganglia output and reduced inhibitory control. Recognizing this pattern is critical, as optimizing medical therapy should be the first step (4).

- **"Peak-Dose" Dystonia/Dyskinesia:** Dystonic postures less commonly emerge or worsen at the peak effect of dopaminergic medication, often as part of biphasic or peak-dose dyskinesias. These are typically of a choreiform pattern but can also have dystonic components, particularly in the limbs or neck [4].

- **Dystonia-Dominant PD:** In some individuals, dystonia, including cervical dystonia, can be a prominent and even initial symptom of PD, sometimes preceding the classic Parkinsonian features. These cases can be challenging to diagnose and may mimic isolated focal dystonias [21].

- **Isolated Cervical Dystonia:** Rarely, patients with idiopathic PD may also have co-occurring primary cervical dystonia, which is not directly related to Parkinsonian pathology or dopaminergic treatment fluctuations. Differentiating this from PD-related dystonia is important for prognosis and treatment planning [21].

3.1.1 Diagnostic considerations for cervical dystonia:

- **Detailed History:** Ascertain the temporal relationship of dystonia with PD onset, medication cycles, and its impact on daily activities and pain.
- **Neurological Examination:** characterization of head posture, direction of pull, the presence of sensory tricks (geste antagoniste), and associated features such as tremor. Dystonic posturing may be temporarily alleviated by sensory tricks, such as a light touch to the chin or head.
- **Response to Dopaminergic Therapy:** A significant improvement in dystonia with levodopa treatment is a strong indicator of its Parkinsonian origin.
- **Exclusion of Other Causes:** Ruling out secondary etiologies of dystonias (e.g., those caused by drugs, structural lesions, or other neurodegenerative disorders) [8].

3.2 Dystonic tremor in PD

Dystonic tremor is a tremor that manifests in a body part affected by dystonia or in association with a dystonic posture. In PD patients, dystonic tremor (DT) can be particularly confusing due to the presence of Parkinsonian rest tremor and, sometimes, co-occurring essential tremor. DT can also be described as "tremor associated with dystonia" if the tremor occurs in a non-dystonic body part.

3.2.1 Characteristics of DT

- **Irregular and Jerky:** DT often appears irregular, jerky, and can be task-specific, differing from the more rhythmic and continuous Parkinsonian rest tremor.
- **Associated with Dystonic Posture:** It is typically present in a body part that is dystonic, such as a head tremor associated with torticollis or a limb tremor accompanying a dystonic limb posture. The tremor may worsen when the patient tries to correct the dystonic posture.
- **Variable Frequency:** The frequency can be variable, often lower than essential tremor but higher than Parkinsonian rest tremor.
- **Sensory Tricks:** Like other dystonias, DT may improve with sensory tricks (geste antagoniste).
- **Activation by Action:** While it can be present at rest, it is often exacerbated by action, posture, or specific movements, blurring the lines with action tremors [22].

3.2.2 Diagnostic considerations for DT

- **Careful Observation:** Observe tremors in different frames (rest, posture, action) and their relationship to any dystonic postures. Look for evidence of co-contraction of agonist and antagonist muscles, which is typical of dystonia.

- **Neurophysiological Studies:** Electromyography can be valuable in differentiating DT. It typically shows co-contraction and irregular burst patterns. In some cases, tremor amplitude varies with dystonic muscle activity, reflecting a tremor–dystonia relationship. This pattern contrasts with the more regular and synchronized bursts observed in Parkinsonian tremor.

- **Response to Treatment:** Although PD-related DT may show partial response to dopaminergic pharmacotherapy, it is often less responsive than Parkinsonian rest tremor. Botulinum toxin injections may help if specific muscles are driving both the dystonia and tremor components.

- **Differentiation from Parkinsonian Rest Tremor:** Parkinsonian resting tremor is typically regular, with a frequency of 4–6 Hz, most prominent at rest, and decreases with voluntary movement. By contrast, DT is often irregular, may vary in frequency, and is strongly linked to dystonic muscle activity.

- **Differentiation from Essential Tremor:** Essential tremor (ET) is typically presented as a postural or action tremor, often bilateral and symmetrical, mostly affecting the upper limbs, head, and voice, usually lacking the prominent dystonic posture seen with DT. However, ET can exhibit mild dystonic features. Misdiagnosis of ET is common, with PD and dystonia often being mistaken for it. Neurophysiological testing and imaging techniques, such as DaT-SPECT, can help distinguish between these tremor syndromes [23, 24].

3.3 Cognitive and psychiatric screening

Psychiatric comorbidities, including anxiety, depression, and body image disturbance, are common in cervical dystonia and dystonic tremor. These factors can significantly affect DBS outcomes, as well as patient satisfaction and postoperative adjustment [25].

4. Conservative therapeutic strategies prior to DBS

Before considering DBS, a range of conservative therapeutic strategies is typically explored for managing cervical dystonia and dystonic tremor in PD. These approaches focus on reducing the symptoms and improving quality of life through pharmacological and non-pharmacological interventions.

4.1 Pharmacological management

Pharmacological treatments are often the first line of defense for both dystonia and tremor in PD.

4.1.1 Dopaminergic medications

For cervical dystonia and dystonic tremor directly linked to PD, optimizing dopaminergic therapy is crucial.

- **Levodopa:** Levodopa, as a precursor of dopamine, is the most effective pharmacological agent for Parkinsonian motor symptoms. Increasing levodopa dosage, changing the frequency of administration, or adding a COMT inhibitor to prolong its effect can be beneficial in the "off-period" dystonia. However, monitoring for potential peak-dose dyskinesias is essential during treatment.

- **Dopamine Agonists:** These medications directly stimulate dopamine receptors and are also beneficial in dystonia, particularly during "off" periods. However, they carry a higher risk of side effects, such as impulse control disorders and hallucinations [26–28].

4.1.2 Botulinum toxin injections

Botulinum toxin injections are considered the gold standard for focal dystonias, including cervical dystonia, and can be highly effective in reducing muscle contractions, abnormal postures, and associated pain [29].

- **Mechanism:** BoNT blocks the release of acetylcholine at the neuromuscular junction, leading to temporary muscle weakness and relaxation.

- **Application:** Injections are targeted directly into the overactive neck muscles responsible for the dystonic posture. The effects typically last for 3–4 months, requiring repeated injections.

- **Benefits for Tremor:** For dystonic tremor, BoNT injections into the dystonic muscles can also help reduce the tremor component, especially if the tremor is highly localized to the dystonic region.

- **Considerations:** Side effects can include dysphagia (difficulty swallowing) or excessive neck weakness, which are typically dose-dependent and temporary [30].

4.1.3 Other oral medications

Various oral medications can be used as adjunctive therapies, although their efficacy is variable and often limited by side effects.

- **Anticholinergics (e.g., Trihexyphenidyl):** Can be effective for dystonia, but side effects such as cognitive impairment, dry mouth, and blurred vision limit their use, especially in older PD patients [31, 32].

- **Benzodiazepines (e.g., Clonazepam):** May help reduce muscle spasms and provide some tremor relief due to their sedative and muscle-relaxant properties but carry risks of drowsiness and dependence [33].

- **Muscle Relaxants (e.g., Baclofen, Tizanidine):** Can be used to alleviate muscle stiffness and spasms in dystonia [31].

- **Beta-blockers (e.g., Propranolol):** Primarily used for essential tremor, they may offer some benefit for dystonic tremor, particularly if there's an overlapping essential tremor component [34].
- **Anticonvulsants (e.g., Levetiracetam, Topiramate):** Occasionally used in refractory dystonia or tremor, but evidence of strong efficacy is limited [34].

4.2 Non-pharmacological management

Non-pharmacological approaches play a supportive role in managing symptoms and improving functional outcomes.

- **Physical and Occupational Therapy:** Can help improve posture, maintain range of motion, reduce pain, and provide training for compensatory strategies. This includes strengthening antagonist muscles, performing stretching exercises, and making ergonomic adjustments [35].
- **Sensory Tricks:** Patients often discover specific sensory stimuli (e.g., touching the chin or the back of the head) that temporarily reduce dystonic spasms. Therapists can help patients identify and utilize these tricks [21].
- **Stress Management and Psychological Support:** Both dystonia and tremor are exacerbated by stress factors. Relaxation exercises, mindfulness, and cognitive-behavioral therapy can be beneficial. Support groups can also provide valuable emotional and practical support [36, 37].
- **Lifestyle Modifications:** Appropriate diet, regular physical activity, optimal sleep, and a commitment to overall well-being contribute to overall health and provide symptomatic relief [37].

Despite these conservative approaches, some patients continue to experience significant and disabling cervical dystonia and dystonic tremor. In such cases, DBS offers an effective and well-established advanced treatment option.

5. DBS: Patient selection and target identification

The decision to proceed with DBS for cervical dystonia and dystonic tremor in the context of PD is a complex one, requiring careful patient selection and precise target identification. This process is typically guided by a multidisciplinary team to ensure optimal outcomes [38].

5.1 Patient selection criteria

Ideal candidates for DBS are those with medically refractory symptoms that significantly impair quality of life, despite optimized pharmacological and non-pharmacological management.

5.1.1 General criteria for DBS in movement disorders

- **Diagnosis Confirmation:** Clear diagnosis of PD, with cervical dystonia and/or dystonic tremor as prominent, disabling symptoms [39].

- **Medically Refractory Symptoms:** Failure to achieve adequate symptom control despite optimal trials of available medications, including levodopa, dopamine agonists, and botulinum toxin administered at appropriate doses and durations, is an important consideration. In patients with "off"-period dystonia, a clear, even if transient, response to levodopa may serve as a positive predictor [38, 39].

- **Impact on Quality of Life:** Significant functional impairment, pain, or social embarrassment due to dystonia and/or tremor [40, 41].

- **Absence of severe cognitive impairment or psychiatric illness:** Depression and anxiety are common and often improve following DBS when mild to moderate. In contrast, severe or uncontrolled psychiatric conditions, including major depression with suicidal ideation, psychosis, or severe dementia, may represent contraindications to surgery. Accordingly, comprehensive neuropsychological assessment is essential [17, 39].

- **Reasonable Surgical Risk:** Patients should be fit for surgery, with no significant comorbidities that would preclude general anesthesia or recovery [17, 39].

- **Realistic Expectations:** Patients and their families must have a clear understanding of the potential benefits and risks of [38].

5.1.2 Specific considerations for cervical dystonia and DT in PD

- **Cervical Dystonia:** Patients with significant pain, severe abnormal postures (torticollis, retrocollis), or functional limitations due to cervical dystonia that do not respond sufficiently to botulinum toxin injections are prime candidates. The presence of "off-period" dystonia is often a good prognostic indicator for GPi DBS [42].

- **Dystonic Tremor:** For disabling dystonic tremor that is poorly controlled by medication or botulinum toxin, DBS can be highly effective. It is important to differentiate it from essential tremor, though both can respond to VIM stimulation [43].

5.2 Target identification

The choice of DBS target is critical and depends largely on the predominant symptoms. The two primary targets for dystonia and tremor are the VIM of the thalamus and the Globus Pallidus Internus. Although the Subthalamic Nucleus (STN) is a less common target for isolated dystonia, it is often chosen for comprehensive PD motor symptoms [17].

5.2.1 Globus pallidus internus

The GPi is the primary surgical target for dystonia, including cervical dystonia, and has shown excellent long-term outcomes [17, 44].

- **Rationale:** The GPi is a key output nucleus of the basal ganglia, and its overactivity is implicated in dystonia pathophysiology. Stimulating the GPi modulates aberrant pallidal activity, thereby reducing dystonic muscle contractions and abnormal postures.

- **Benefits:** GPi DBS can significantly improve dystonia severity, reduce pain, and enhance quality of life. The benefits for dystonia are often delayed, taking several months to achieve maximal effect. It can also improve other Parkinsonian symptoms, particularly dyskinesias.

- **Considerations:** While effective for dystonia, GPi stimulation may have less direct impact on tremor compared to VIM stimulation, although some tremor improvement can occur, especially if it's secondary to the dystonia.

5.2.2 Ventral intermediate nucleus of the thalamus

The VIM is the established target for tremor suppression, including essential tremor and Parkinsonian tremor, and it is also effective for dystonic tremor [22].

- **Rationale:** The VIM is part of the cerebello-thalamo-cortical circuit, which is central to tremor generation. VIM stimulation disrupts the pathological oscillatory activity within this circuit, leading to tremor attenuation.

- **Benefits:** VIM DBS provides robust and often immediate tremor suppression. It can be particularly effective for disabling dystonic tremor, which has a significant oscillatory component.

- **Considerations:** While highly effective for tremor, VIM stimulation typically has little to no direct effect on the underlying dystonic postures or the pain associated with dystonia. Therefore, if cervical dystonia is the predominant and most disabling symptom, GPi is generally preferred.

5.2.3 Subthalamic nucleus

In PD, the STN represents the most frequently selected target for achieving broad motor symptom control, leading to significant improvements in bradykinesia, rigidity, and tremor, while enabling reductions in dopaminergic medication [17].

- **Rationale:** STN stimulation normalizes the aberrant activity within the basal ganglia network.

- **Benefits for Dystonia/Tremor in PD:** STN DBS can improve both Parkinsonian tremor and "off-period" dystonia associated with PD. However, for primary or severe isolated dystonia, GPi is generally considered superior.

- **Considerations:** STN DBS can sometimes induce or worsen dyskinesias or psychiatric side effects if not carefully programmed. For isolated cervical dystonia, STN DBS is generally not the first choice.

5.2.4 Dual-targeting or combined approaches

In complex cases with severe, medically intractable cervical dystonia and disabling dystonic tremor, a combined approach might be considered, such as bilateral GPi for dystonia and unilateral VIM for a particularly debilitating tremor, or even sequential targeting. However, these approaches should be tailored to individual patient characteristics due to their increased technical complexity and potential risks [45].

5.3 Surgical planning and implantation

Precision in surgical planning is paramount. Advanced imaging techniques, including MRI and CT, are used to create a detailed map of the brain and guide electrode placement. Intraoperative neurophysiology, such as microelectrode recording, helps confirm the target location by listening to the electrical activity of individual neurons, ensuring the electrode is within the optimal therapeutic zone. Some centers also utilize awake surgery, with patient cooperation, to assess immediate stimulation effects on symptoms and side effects [46, 47].

6. Programming paradigms and postoperative management

Effective programming of DBS devices is as crucial as accurate lead placement for optimizing therapeutic outcomes in cervical dystonia and dystonic tremor in PD. Postoperative management involves a systematic approach to adjusting stimulation parameters to achieve maximal symptom control while minimizing side effects [48].

6.1 Principles of DBS programming

DBS devices deliver continuous electrical pulses, and programming involves adjusting several parameters [49]:

- **Contact Selection:** Each lead typically has multiple electrodes (contacts). Programmers select which contacts or combinations of contacts (e.g., monopolar, bipolar, multipolar) will deliver the current. Directional leads further enhance this by allowing current steering, directing stimulation away from adjacent structures that could cause side effects [50].

- **Amplitude:** This determines the strength of the electrical pulse. It is gradually increased until therapeutic benefits are observed, or side effects appear.

- **Pulse Width:** The duration of each electrical pulse. Longer pulse widths can recruit more tissue but may also increase the risk of side effects [47].

- **Frequency:** The number of pulses per second. High frequencies (typically 130–185 Hz) are commonly used for tremor and dystonia, but lower frequencies may be explored in some cases, particularly in dystonia [51].

6.2 Programming for cervical dystonia

Programming for dystonia, especially cervical dystonia, presents unique challenges compared to other movement disorders.

- **Delayed Therapeutic Effect:** Unlike Parkinsonian tremor, which often responds acutely to stimulation, the full therapeutic benefit for dystonia can be significantly delayed, sometimes taking several weeks to months to become apparent. This necessitates patience and a structured, gradual approach to programming [47].

- **Initial Settings and Adjustments:** Stimulation is typically initiated a few weeks post-surgery (e.g., 2-4 weeks). Initial settings might include a low voltage (e.g., 1.0-1.5 V), high frequency (e.g., 130 Hz), and a pulse width around 60 μs [46].

- **Systematic Increments:** Amplitude is usually increased gradually over weeks or months. Clinicians observe both symptom improvement and the emergence of side effects such as dysarthria, muscle contractions, or gaze deviation. If side effects occur, the amplitude is decreased or the contact configuration is changed (e.g., from monopolar to bipolar) [52].

- **Contact Optimization:** Programmers prioritize contacts that offer the best therapeutic window (maximal benefit with minimal side effects). Software packages can assist in visualizing the volume of tissue activated, aiding in contact selection. Focusing on the deepest contacts in the posteroventral pallidum often provides the most benefit [52].

- **Adjuvant Therapies:** Even after DBS, some patients with cervical dystonia may continue to benefit from adjuvant oral medications or botulinum toxin injections to optimize symptom control [53].

6.3 Programming for dystonic tremor

Programming for dystonic tremor shares similarities with programming for essential tremor or Parkinsonian tremor, given the shared neural circuits involved in tremor generation [54].

- **Immediate Effect:** Tremor suppression is often more immediate compared to dystonia, making it easier to assess the acute effects of stimulation adjustments [47].

- **Standard Parameters:** High-frequency stimulation (e.g., 130–185 Hz) is commonly used. Pulse widths are typically in the range of 60–100 μs, and voltage is titrated to achieve tremor control without inducing side effects [48, 51].

- **Side Effect Management:** Potential side effects, such as dysarthria, paresthesias, or gait disturbances, are carefully monitored. Adjustments to voltage, pulse width, or contact selection can help mitigate these side effects [17].

- **Multitarget Programming:** In cases of dual-target DBS (e.g., GPi + VIM or STN + VIM), each target is programmed independently, but the overall effect on both dystonia and tremor must be considered, often requiring a collaborative approach to balance therapeutic outcomes [43, 55].

6.4 Postoperative management and follow-up

- Regular follow-up visits are essential for long-term DBS care in order to assess patient improvement and adjust stimulation parameters.

- **Initial Intensive Phase:** The first few months post-implantation typically involve more frequent programming sessions as the patient adapts to stimulation and the full effects of therapy unfold [56, 57].

- **Ongoing Adjustment:** Parameters may need to be adjusted over time due to disease progression, changes in medication, or the development of new symptoms or side effects [39, 46].

- **Multidisciplinary Approach:** A multidisciplinary team, including neurologists, neurosurgeons, nurses, and sometimes neuropsychologists and physical therapists, is essential for comprehensive postoperative care. This team evaluates not only motor symptoms but also cognitive, psychiatric, and quality-of-life aspects [17, 58].

- **Patient Education:** Educating patients about their device, how to identify side effects, and when to seek assistance is crucial for successful long-term management [49, 59].

7. Personalized neuromodulation, adaptive DBS, and emerging technologies

Personalized neuromodulation represents the evolution from one-size-fits-all continuous DBS to patient-specific therapies that adapt to individual neural dynamics and clinical states. aDBS, also known as closed-loop DBS, uses real-time biomarkers, such as local field potentials or electromyography, to dynamically modulate stimulation parameters, optimizing efficacy while minimizing side effects and battery consumption [60, 61].

In PD with dystonia or tremor, β -band LFPs (13–30 Hz) from the STN have emerged as promising biomarkers for motor state detection, correlating with symptom severity and responding to stimulation [62]. Although primarily validated in PD, pathological oscillations in dystonic networks suggest potential extension to cervical dystonia and dystonic tremor. Algorithms include single/dual-threshold, proportional control, or machine learning-based reinforcement learning to titrate stimulation.

Emerging technologies further enable precision:

- **Directional Leads and Current Steering:** Segmented electrodes allow field shaping to target specific circuits, such as the dentato-rubro-thalamic tract, thereby expanding the therapeutic window [50, 63].
- **Chronic Sensing Devices:** Systems like Percept PC enable home-based LFP monitoring for biomarker-guided adjustments [50].
- **AI-Enhanced Programming:** Data-driven models automate parameter optimization, reducing clinicians' burden [64].
- **Connectomics and Robotics:** Diffusion tensor imaging refines trajectory planning; robotic assistance improves accuracy [65].
- **Remote Programming:** Wireless connectivity facilitates telemedicine, accelerating optimization [66].

These innovations promise tailored therapy for heterogeneous phenotypes, such as dystonic tremor.

8. Challenges and limitations

Despite advances, DBS for cervical dystonia and dystonic tremor still faces hurdles.

- **Heterogeneity and Response Variability:** Delayed dystonia benefits (weeks–months) complicate acute assessment; non-responders (~20%–30%) challenge prediction [67].
- **Programming Complexity:** Requires expertise; side effects (e.g., dysarthria) demand iterative adjustments [68].
- **Biomarker Gaps:** Dystonia-specific signals lag behind PD β -bursts [69].
- **Complications:** Infection (~2%–5%), hardware failure, battery replacement; long-term efficacy wanes in some cases [43].
- **Access and Expertise:** Limited to specialized centers; pediatric/young-onset cases add complexity [70].

Multidisciplinary care and controlled clinical trials are essential to improve outcomes and guide future DBS strategies.

9. Conclusion

Cervical dystonia and dystonic tremor represent complex and often debilitating motor phenotypes within the broader spectrum of PD, significantly impacting patients' quality of life. These conditions challenge traditional diagnostic categories and highlight the limitations of approaches focused solely on dopaminergic deficiency or isolated motor nuclei. As clinical experience and neuroscientific understanding have expanded, it has become increasingly clear that these phenotypes arise from dysfunction within distributed motor networks rather than from a single pathological node [8].

DBS has emerged as an established and highly effective neurosurgical intervention for these medically refractory symptoms. The choice of DBS target is crucial and phenotype-driven: the Globus Pallidus Internus is the preferred target for cervical dystonia and dystonia-dominant Parkinsonian features, offering significant and sustained improvements in motor symptoms, pain, and quality of life. For dystonic tremor, the VIM of the thalamus provides robust tremor suppression, though its effect on underlying dystonic posturing is limited. In cases of severe mixed symptoms, dual-targeting approaches are being explored to address both dystonia and tremor components more comprehensively [42, 43, 58, 71].

The success of DBS relies on a meticulous, multidisciplinary approach encompassing patient selection, precise surgical implantation, and nuanced postoperative care. While conventional continuous DBS remains effective, the field is rapidly advancing toward more personalized and adaptive strategies. aDBS and closed-loop systems, which utilize real-time neural biomarkers to dynamically adjust stimulation, hold immense promise for optimizing therapeutic effects, reducing side effects, and conserving battery life. Further developments in connectomic targeting, AI-enhanced programming, and hardware innovations such as directional leads are poised to refine neuromodulation, making it more tailored and accessible [1, 17, 69, 72].

Despite considerable progress, challenges remain, including the inherent heterogeneity of dystonia and tremor, the complexity of programming, and the need for more specific biomarkers. Continued research into the precise mechanisms of DBS and the underlying pathophysiology of these conditions will be vital. The ultimate goal is to move from symptom-based intervention to truly personalized, network-informed therapy that aligns with each patient's unique neural signatures, thereby enhancing long-term outcomes and improving the lives of individuals with cervical dystonia and dystonic tremor in PD [1, 68].

Acknowledgments

The authors declare that no external funding was received for this work. The authors alone are responsible for the content and writing of this chapter.

Materials and methods

Artificial intelligence (AI)-based language tools were used to improve the clarity and readability of the manuscript. The authors reviewed and approved the final version. (GEMINI 3)

Conflict of Interest

The authors declare no conflict of interest.

Author details

Akın Akakın*, Emre Ünal and Abdullah Andaç
Neurosurgery Department, Bahçeşehir University Medical Faculty, Istanbul, Türkiye

*Address all correspondence to: drakinakakin@yahoo.com

References

[1] Krauss JK, Lipsman N, Aziz T, Boutet A, Brown P, Chang JW, Davidson B, Grill WM, Hariz MI, Horn A, Schulder M, Mammis A, Tass PA, Volkmann J, Lozano AM. Technology of deep brain stimulation: Current status and future directions. Nature Reviews Neurology. 2021;**17**(2):75–87. DOI: 10.1038/s41582-020-00426-z

[2] Jankovic J, Tan EK. Parkinson's disease: Etiopathogenesis and treatment. Journal of Neurology, Neurosurgery & Psychiatry. 2020;**91**(8):795–808. DOI: 10.1136/jnnp-2019-322338

[3] Tolosa E, Garrido A, Scholz SW, Poewe W. Challenges in the diagnosis of Parkinson's disease. The Lancet Neurology. 2021;**20**(5):385–397. DOI: 10.1016/S1474-4422(21)00030-2

[4] Tolosa E, Compta Y. Dystonia in Parkinson's disease. Journal of Neurology. 2006;**253**(Suppl 7):VII7–13. DOI: 10.1007/s00415-006-7003-6

[5] Liu X, Guang J, Glowinsky S, Abadi H, Arkadir D, Linetsky E, Abu Snineh M, León JF, Israel Z, Wang W, Bergman H. Subthalamic nucleus input-output dynamics are correlated with Parkinson's burden and treatment efficacy. Npj Parkinson's Disease. 2024;**10**(1):117. DOI: 10.1038/s41531-024-00737-8

[6] Eleopra R, Rinaldo S, Devigili G, Mondani M, D'Auria S, Golfrè Andreasi N, Skrap M, Lettieri C. Globus pallidus internus deep brain stimulation using frame-based vs. frameless stereotaxy in dystonia: A single-center experience. Frontiers in Neurology. 2021;**12**:643757. DOI: 10.3389/fneur.2021.643757

[7] Liu B, Xu J, Feng Z, Hui R, Zhang Y, Liu D, Chang Q, Yu X, Mao Z. One-pass deep brain stimulation of subthalamic nucleus and ventral intermediate nucleus for levodopa-resistant tremor-dominant Parkinson's disease. Frontiers in Aging Neuroscience. 2023;**15**:1289183. DOI: 10.3389/fnagi.2023.1289183

[8] Defazio G, Belvisi D, Comella C, Hallett M, Jinnah HA, Cimino P, Latorre A, Mascia MM, Rocchi L, Gigante AF, Ercoli T, Berardelli A. Validation of a guideline to reduce variability in diagnosing cervical dystonia. Journal of Neurology. 2023;**270**(5):2606–2612. DOI: 10.1007/s00415-023-11585-6

[9] Merola A, Singh J, Reeves K, Changizi B, Goetz S, Rossi L, Pallavaram S, Carcieri S, Harel N, Shaikhouni A, Sammartino F, Krishna V, Verhagen L, Dalm B. New frontiers for deep brain stimulation: Directionality, sensing technologies, remote programming, robotic stereotactic assistance, asleep procedures, and connectomics. Frontiers in Neurology. 2021;**12**:694747. DOI: 10.3389/fneur.2021.694747

[10] Di Biasio F, Marchese R, Abbruzzese G, Baldi O, Esposito M, Silvestre F, Tescione G, Berardelli A, Fabbrini G, Ferrazzano G, Pellicciari R, Eleopra R, Devigili G, Bono F, Santangelo D, Bertolasi L, Altavista MC, Moschella V, Barone P, Erro R, Albanese A, Scaglione C, Liguori R, Cotelli MS, Cossu G, Ceravolo R, Coletti Moja M, Zibetti M, Pisani A, Petracca M,

Tinazzi M, Maderna L, Girlanda P, Magistrelli L, Misceo S, Romano M, Minafra B, Modugno N, Aguggia M, Cassano D, Defazio G, Avanzino L. Motor and sensory features of cervical dystonia subtypes: Data from the italian dystonia registry. Frontiers in Neurology. 2020;**11**:906. DOI: 10.3389/fneur.2020.00906

[11] Koeglsperger T, Palleis C, Hell F, Mehrkens JH, Bötzel K. deep brain stimulation programming for movement disorders: Current concepts and evidence-based strategies. Frontiers in Neurology. 2019;**10**:410. DOI: 10.3389/fneur.2019.00410

[12] Neychev VK, Gross RE, Lehéricy S, Hess EJ, Jinnah HA. The functional neuroanatomy of dystonia. Neurobiology of Disease. 2011;**42**(2):185–201. DOI: 10.1016/j.nbd.2011.01.026

[13] Bologna M, Paparella G, Colella D, Cannavacciuolo A, Angelini L, Alunni-Fegatelli D, Guerra A, Berardelli A. Is there evidence of bradykinesia in essential tremor? European Journal of Neurology. 2020;**27**(8):1501–1509. DOI: 10.1111/ene.14312

[14] Wichmann T, DeLong MR. Deep Brain Stimulation for Movement Disorders of Basal Ganglia Origin: Restoring Function or Functionality? Neurotherapeutics: The Journal of the American Society for Experimental NeuroTherapeutics. 2016;**13**(2):264–283. DOI: 10.1007/s13311-016-0426-6

[15] Brüggemann N. Contemporary functional neuroanatomy and pathophysiology of dystonia. Journal of Neural Transmission. 2021;**128**(4):499–508. DOI: 10.1007/s00702-021-02299-y

[16] Higginbotham L, Scorr LM, Parra SP, Sommerfeld B, Jinnah HA, Factor SA. Prevalence and clinical features of cervical dystonia in Parkinson's disease. Parkinsonism & Related Disorders. 2024;**127**:107114. DOI: 10.1016/j.parkreldis.2024.107114

[17] Hariz M, Blomstedt P. Deep brain stimulation for Parkinson's disease. Journal of Internal Medicine. 2022;**292**(5):764–778. DOI: 10.1111/joim.13541

[18] Ellis EG, Meyer GM, Kaasinen V, Corp DT, Pavese N, Reich MM, Joutsa J. Multimodal neuroimaging to characterize symptom-specific networks in movement disorders. Npj Parkinson's Disease. 2024;**10**(1):154. DOI: 10.1038/s41531-024-00774-3

[19] Thomsen M, Lange LM, Zech M, Lohmann K. Genetics and Pathogenesis of Dystonia. Annual Review of Pathology: Mechanisms of Disease. 2024;**19**:99–131. DOI: 10.1146/annurev-pathmechdis-051122-110756

[20] Singh A. Oscillatory activity in the cortico-basal ganglia-thalamic neural circuits in Parkinson's disease. European Journal of Neuroscience. 2018;**48**(8):2869–2878. DOI: 10.1111/ejn.13853

[21] Albanese A, Bhatia KP, Cardoso F, Comella C, Defazio G, Fung VSC, Hallett M, Jankovic J, Jinnah HA, Kaji R, Krauss JK, Lang A, Tan EK, Tijssen MAJ, Vidailhet M. Isolated Cervical Dystonia: Diagnosis and Classification. Movement Disorders. 2023;**38**(8):1367–1378. DOI: 10.1002/mds.29387

[22] Bhatia KP, Bain P, Bajaj N, Elble RJ, Hallett M, Louis ED, Raethjen J, Stamelou M, Testa CM, Deuschl G. Tremor task force of the international parkinson and movement disorder

society. Consensus statement on the classification of tremors. From the task force on tremor of the International Parkinson and Movement Disorder Society. Journal of Neural Transmission. 2018;**33**(1):75–87. DOI: 10.1002/mds.27121

[23] Chen W, Hopfner F, Becktepe JS, Deuschl G. Rest tremor revisited: Parkinson's disease and other disorders. Translational Neurodegeneration. 2017;**6**:16. DOI: 10.1186/s40035-017-0086-4

[24] Quattrone A, Nisticò R, Morelli M, Arabia G, Crasà M, Vescio B, Mechelli A, Cascini GL, Quattrone A. Rest tremor pattern predicts DaTscan (^{123}I-Ioflupane) result in tremulous disorders. Movement Disorders. 2021;**36**(12):2964–2966. DOI: 10.1002/mds.28797

[25] Bailey GA, Martin E, Peall KJ. Cognitive and Neuropsychiatric Impairment in Dystonia. Current Neurology and Neuroscience Reports. 2022;**22**(11):699–708. DOI: 10.1007/s11910-022-01233-3

[26] Connolly BS, Lang AE. Pharmacological treatment of Parkinson disease: A review. JAMA. 2014;**311**(16):1670–1683. DOI: 10.1001/jama.2014.3654

[27] Höllerhage M, Becktepe J, Classen J, Deuschl G, Ebersbach G, Hopfner F, Lingor P, Löhle M, Maaß S, Pötter-Nerger M, Odin P, Woitalla D, Parkinson's Guidelines Group G, Trenkwalder C, Höglinger GU. Pharmacotherapy of motor symptoms in early and mid-stage Parkinson's disease: Guideline "Parkinson's disease" of the German Society of Neurology. Journal of Neurology. 2024;**271**(11):7071–7101. DOI: 10.1007/s00415-024-12632-6

[28] LeWitt PA. Levodopa therapy for Parkinson's disease: Pharmacokinetics and pharmacodynamics. Movement Disorders. 2015;**30**(1):64–72. DOI: 10.1002/mds.26082

[29] Simpson DM, Hallett M, Ashman EJ, Comella CL, Green MW, Gronseth GS, Armstrong MJ, Gloss D, Potrebic S, Jankovic J, Karp BP, Naumann M, So YT, Yablon SA. Practice guideline update summary: Botulinum neurotoxin for the treatment of blepharospasm, cervical dystonia, adult spasticity, and headache [RETIRED]: Report of the Guideline Development Subcommittee of the American Academy of Neurology. Neurology. 2016;**86**(19):1818–1826. DOI: 10.1212/WNL.0000000000002560

[30] Albanese A, Abbruzzese G, Dressler D, Duzynski W, Khatkova S, Marti MJ, Mir P, Montecucco C, Moro E, Pinter M, Relja M, Roze E, Skogseid IM, Timerbaeva S, Tzoulis C. Practical guidance for CD management involving treatment of botulinum toxin: A consensus statement. Journal of Neurology. 2015;**262**(10):2201–2213. DOI: 10.1007/s00415-015-7703-x

[31] Albanese A, Barnes MP, Bhatia KP, Fernandez-Alvarez E, Filippini G, Gasser T, Krauss JK, Newton A, Rektor I, Savoiardo M, Valls-Solè J. A systematic review on the diagnosis and treatment of primary (idiopathic) dystonia and dystonia plus syndromes: Report of an EFNS/MDS-ES Task Force. European Journal of Neurology. 2006;**13**(5):433–444. DOI: 10.1111/j.1468-1331.2006.01537.x

[32] Lange LM, Junker J, Loens S, Baumann H, Olschewski L, Schaake S, Madoev H, Petkovic S, Kuhnke N, Kasten M, Westenberger A, Domingo A,

Marras C, König IR, Camargos S, Ozelius LJ, Klein C, Lohmann K. Genotype–Phenotype Relations for Isolated Dystonia Genes: MDSGene Systematic Review. Movement Disorders. 2021;**36**(5):1086–1103. DOI: 10.1002/mds.28485

[33] Fasano A, Bove F, Lang AE. The treatment of dystonic tremor: A systematic review. Journal of Neurology, Neurosurgery & Psychiatry. 2014;**85**(7):759–769. DOI: 10.1136/jnnp-2013-305532

[34] Ferreira JJ, Mestre TA, Lyons KE, Benito-León J, Tan EK, Abbruzzese G, Hallett M, Haubenberger D, Elble R, Deuschl G. MDS Task Force on Tremor and the MDS Evidence Based Medicine Committee. MDS evidence-based review of treatments for essential tremor. Movement Disorders. 2019;**34**(7):950–958. DOI: 10.1002/mds.27700

[35] Girach A, Vinagre Aragon A, Zis P. Quality of life in idiopathic dystonia: A systematic review. Journal of Neurology. 2019;**266**(12):2897–2906. DOI: 10.1007/s00415-018-9119-x

[36] Maione R, Formica C, Quartarone A, Lo Buono V. the impact of non-motor symptoms on quality of life in cervical dystonia. Journal of Clinical Medicine. 2023;**12**(14):4663. DOI: 10.3390/jcm12144663

[37] Koptielow J, Szyłak E, Szewczyk-Roszczenko O, Roszczenko P, Kochanowicz J, Kułakowska A, Chorąży M. Genetic Update and Treatment for Dystonia. International Journal of Molecular Sciences. 2024;**25**(7):3571. DOI: 10.3390/ijms25073571

[38] Wagle Shukla A, Bange M, Muthuraman M. Patient, target, device, and program selection for DBS in Parkinson's disease: Advancing toward precision care. Npj Parkinson's Disease. 2025;**11**(1):195. DOI: 10.1038/s41531-025-01015-x

[39] Deuschl G, Antonini A, Costa J, Śmiłowska K, Berg D, Corvol JC, Fabbrini G, Ferreira J, Foltynie T, Mir P, Schrag A, Seppi K, Taba P, Ruzicka E, Selikhova M, Henschke N, Villanueva G, Moro E. European Academy of Neurology/Movement Disorder Society-European Section Guideline on the Treatment of Parkinson's Disease: I. Movement Disorders. 2022;**37**(7):1360–1374. DOI: 10.1002/mds.29066

[40] Mahlknecht P, Foltynie T, Limousin P, Poewe W. How does deep brain stimulation change the course of parkinson's disease? Movement Disorders. 2022;**37**(8):1581–1592. DOI: 10.1002/mds.29052

[41] Schuepbach WMM, Tonder L, Schnitzler A, Krack P, Rau J, Hartmann A, Hälbig TD, Pineau F, Falk A, Paschen L, Paschen S, Volkmann J, Dafsari HS, Barbe MT, Fink GR, Kühn A, Kupsch A, Schneider GH, Seigneuret E, Fraix V, Kistner A, Chaynes PP, Ory-Magne F, Brefel-Courbon C, Vesper J, Wojtecki L, Derrey S, Maltête D, Damier P, Derkinderen P, Sixel-Döring F, Trenkwalder C, Gharabaghi A, Wächter T, Weiss D, Pinsker MO, Regis JM, Witjas T, Thobois S, Mertens P, Knudsen K, Schade-Brittinger C, Houeto JL, Agid Y, Vidailhet M, Timmermann L, Deuschl G. EARLYSTIM study group. Quality of life predicts outcome of deep brain stimulation in early Parkinson disease. Neurology. 2019;**92**(10):e1109–e1120. DOI: 10.1212/WNL.0000000000007037. Erratum in: Neurology. 2019 Jun 11;92(24):1166. doi:

10.1212/WNL.0000000000007420. PMID: 30737338; PMCID: PMC6442017

[42] Krack P, Volkmann J, Tinkhauser G, Deuschl G. Deep brain stimulation in movement disorders: From experimental surgery to evidence-based therapy. Movement Disorders. 2019;**34**(12):1795–1810. DOI: 10.1002/mds.27860

[43] Tsuboi T, Jabarkheel Z, Zeilman PR, Barabas MJ, Foote KD, Okun MS, Wagle Shukla A. Longitudinal follow-up with VIM thalamic deep brain stimulation for dystonic or essential tremor. Neurology. 2020;**94**(10):e1073–e1084. DOI: 10.1212/WNL.0000000000008875

[44] Panyakaew P, Phuenpathom W, Bhidayasiri R, Hallett M. Bedside clinical assessment of patients with common upper limb tremor and algorithmic approach. Asian Biomedicine. 2024;**18**(2):37–52. DOI: 10.2478/abm-2024-0008

[45] Ramirez-Zamora A, Giordano J, Boyden ES, Gradinaru V, Gunduz A, Starr PA, Sheth SA, McIntyre CC, Fox MD, Vitek J, Vedam-Mai V, Akbar U, Almeida L, Bronte-Stewart HM, Mayberg HS, Pouratian N, Gittis AH, Singer AC, Creed MC, Lazaro-Munoz G, Richardson M, Rossi MA, Cendejas-Zaragoza L, D'Haese PF, Chiong W, Gilron R, Chizeck H, Ko A, Baker KB, Wagenaar J, Harel N, Deeb W, Foote KD, Okun MS. Proceedings of the Sixth Deep Brain Stimulation Think Tank Modulation of Brain Networks and Application of Advanced Neuroimaging, Neurophysiology, and Optogenetics. Frontiers in Neuroscience. 2019;**13**:936. DOI: 10.3389/fnins.2019.00936

[46] Capelle HH, Krauss JK. Neuromodulation in dystonia: Current aspects of deep brain stimulation. Neuromodulation: Technology at the Neural Interface. 2009;**12**(1):8–21. DOI: 10.1111/j.1525-1403.2009.00183.x

[47] Fan H, Zheng Z, Yin Z, Zhang J, Lu G. Deep brain stimulation treating dystonia: A systematic review of targets, body distributions and etiology classifications. Frontiers in Human Neuroscience. 2021;**15**:757579. DOI: 10.3389/fnhum.2021.757579

[48] Smeets S, Boogers A, Van Bogaert T, Peeters J, McLaughlin M, Nuttin B, Theys T, Vandenberghe W, De Vloo P. Deep brain stimulation with short versus conventional pulse width in Parkinson's disease and essential tremor: A systematic review and meta-analysis. Brain Stimulation. 2024;**17**(1):71–82. DOI: 10.1016/j.brs.2023.12.013

[49] Nagel JM, Wolf ME, Blahak C, Runge J, Schrader C, Dressler D, Saryyeva A, Krauss JK. Thalamic deep brain stimulation for dystonic head tremor: A long-term study of 18 patients. Movement Disorders Clinical Practice. 2026;**13**(1):131–141. DOI: 10.1002/mdc3.70266

[50] Lo Faso V, Schisano L, Remore LG, Tariciotti L, Fiore G, Valcamonica G, Borellini L, Cogiamanian F, D'Ammando A, Pirola E, Ampollini A, Marfia G, Locatelli M. Deep brain stimulation in parkinson disease: A switch for On/Off Dystonia. World Neurosurgery. 2025;**194**:123438. DOI: 10.1016/j.wneu.2024.11.021

[51] Kuncel AM, Cooper SE, Wolgamuth BR, Clyde MA, Snyder SA, EB Jr M, Rezai AR, Grill WM. Clinical response to varying the stimulus

parameters in deep brain stimulation for essential tremor. Movement Disorders. 2006;**21**(11):1920–1928. DOI: 10.1002/mds.21087

[52] Fox MD, Alterman RL. Brain stimulation for torsion dystonia. JAMA Neurology. 2015;**72**(6):713–719. DOI: 10.1001/jamaneurol.2015.51

[53] Qiu Y, Xue T, Bai Y, Han C, Xie M, Teng H, Yin Z, Chen Z, Zhang J, Wang Z. Comparison of different surgical strategies for cervical dystonia: Evidence from Bayesian network analysis. European Journal of Neurology. 2025;**32**(1):e16527. DOI: 10.1111/ene.16527

[54] Tsuboi T, Wong JK, Eisinger RS, Okromelidze L, Burns MR, Ramirez-Zamora A, Almeida L, Wagle Shukla A, Foote KD, Okun MS, Grewal SS, Middlebrooks EH. Comparative connectivity correlates of dystonic and essential tremor deep brain stimulation. Brain. 2021;**144**(6):1774–1786. DOI: 10.1093/brain/awab074. Erratum in: Brain. 2021 Sep 4;144(8)e71. doi: 10.1093/brain/awab192. PMID: 33889943

[55] Paoli D, Mills R, Brechany U, Pavese N, Nicholson C. DBS in tremor with dystonia: VIM, GPi or both? A review of the literature and considerations from a single-center experience. Journal of Neurology. 2023;**270**(4):2217–2229. DOI: 10.1007/s00415-023-11569-6

[56] Gharabaghi A, Groppa S, Navas-Garcia M, Schnitzler A, Muñoz-Delgado L, Marshall VL, Karl J, Zhang L, Alvarez R, Feldman MS, Soileau MJ, Luo L, Zauber SE, Walter BL, Wu C, Lei H, Herz DM, Chung MH, Pathak Y, Blomme B, Cheeran B, Luca C, Weiss D. Accelerated symptom improvement in Parkinson's disease via remote internet-based optimization of deep brain stimulation therapy: A randomized controlled multicenter trial. Communications Medicine. 2025;**5**(1):31. DOI: 10.1038/s43856-025-00744-7

[57] Gharabaghi A, Groppa S, Casas E, Schnitzler A, Muñoz-Delgado L, Marshall VL, Karl J, Zhang L, Alvarez R, Feldman MS, Soileau MJ, Luo L, Walter BL, Wu C, Lei H, Herz DM, Nanduri D, Salazar CA, Luca C, Weiss D. Real-world multicenter assessment of sustained clinical outcomes after digital deep brain stimulation. Npj Digital Medicine. 2026;**9**(1):133. DOI: 10.1038/s41746-025-02315-5

[58] Lozano AM, Lipsman N, Bergman H, Brown P, Chabardes S, Chang JW, Matthews K, McIntyre CC, Schlaepfer TE, Schulder M, Temel Y, Volkmann J, Krauss JK. Deep brain stimulation: Current challenges and future directions. Nature Reviews Neurology. 2019;**15**(3):148–160. DOI: 10.1038/s41582-018-0128-2

[59] J FADS, du Montcel S T, Gargiulo M, Behar C, Montel S, Hergueta T, Navarro S, Belaid H, Cloitre P, Karachi C, Mallet L, Welter ML. Tackling psychosocial maladjustment in Parkinson's disease patients following subthalamic deep-brain stimulation: A randomised clinical trial. PLoS One. 2017;**12**(4):e0174512. DOI: 10.1371/journal.pone.0174512

[60] Neumann WJ, Horn A, Kühn AA. Insights and opportunities for deep brain stimulation as a brain circuit intervention. Trends in Neurosciences. 2023;**46**(6):472–487. DOI: 10.1016/j.tins.2023.03.009

[61] Guidetti M, Marceglia S, Loh A, Harmsen IE, Meoni S, Foffani G,

Lozano AM, Moro E, Volkmann J, Priori A. Clinical perspectives of adaptive deep brain stimulation. Brain Stimulation. 2021;**14**(5):1238–1247. DOI: 10.1016/j.brs.2021.07.063

[62] van Wijk BCM, de Bie RMA, Beudel M. A systematic review of local field potential physiomarkers in Parkinson's disease: From clinical correlations to adaptive deep brain stimulation algorithms. Journal of Neurology. 2023;**270**(2):1162–1177. DOI: 10.1007/s00415-022-11388-1

[63] Hvingelby V, Khalil F, Massey F, Hoyningen A, Xu SS, Candelario-mckeown J, Akram H, Foltynie T, Limousin P, Zrinzo L, Krüger MT. Directional deep brain stimulation electrodes in Parkinson's disease: Meta-analysis and systematic review of the literature. Journal of Neurology, Neurosurgery & Psychiatry. 2025;**96**(2):188–198. DOI: 10.1136/jnnp-2024-333947

[64] Oliveira AM, Coelho L, Carvalho E, Ferreira-Pinto MJ, Vaz R, Aguiar P. Machine learning for adaptive deep brain stimulation in Parkinson's disease: Closing the loop. Journal of Neurology. 2023;**270**(11):5313–5326. DOI: 10.1007/s00415-023-11873-1

[65] Neudorfer C, Butenko K, Oxenford S, Rajamani N, Achtzehn J, Goede L, Hollunder B, Ríos AS, Hart L, Tasserie J, Fernando KB, Nguyen TAK, Al-Fatly B, Vissani M, Fox M, Richardson RM, van Rienen U, Kühn AA, Husch AD, Opri E, Dembek T, Li N, Horn A. Lead-DBS v3.0: Mapping deep brain stimulation effects to local anatomy and global networks. Neuroimage. 2023;**268**:119862. DOI: 10.1016/j.neuroimage.2023.119862

[66] Swinnen BEKS, Buijink AW, Piña-Fuentes D, de Bie RMA, Beudel M. Diving into the subcortex: The potential of chronic subcortical sensing for unravelling basal ganglia function and optimization of deep brain stimulation. Neuroimage. 2022;**254**:119147. DOI: 10.1016/j.neuroimage.2022.119147

[67] Raghu ALB, Eraifej J, Sarangmat N, Stein J, FitzGerald JJ, Payne S, Aziz TZ, Green AL. Pallido-putaminal connectivity predicts outcomes of deep brain stimulation for cervical dystonia. Brain. 2021;**144**(12):3589–3596. DOI: 10.1093/brain/awab280

[68] Lange F, Soares C, Roothans J, Raimundo R, Eldebakey H, Weigl B, Peach R, Daniels C, Musacchio T, Volkmann J, Rosas MJ, Reich MM. Machine versus physician-based programming of deep brain stimulation in isolated dystonia: A feasibility study. Brain Stimulation. 2023;**16**(4):1105–1111. DOI: 10.1016/j.brs.2023.06.018

[69] Johnson KA, Coutinho PB, Sarmento FP, Vo E, Wong JK, Hilliard JD, Foote KD, de Hemptinne C. Pallidal evoked resonant neural activity as a candidate biomarker for deep brain stimulation in dystonia. Movement Disorders: Official Journal of the Movement Disorder Society. 2025;**41**:709–718. DOI: 10.1002/mds.70129

[70] Lee DJ, Lozano CS, Dallapiazza RF, Lozano AM. Current and future directions of deep brain stimulation for neurological and psychiatric disorders. Journal of Neurosurgery. 2019;**131**(2):333–342. DOI: 10.3171/2019.4.JNS181761

[71] Parker T, Raghu ALB, FitzGerald JJ, Green AL, Aziz TZ. Multitarget deep brain stimulation for

clinically complex movement disorders. Journal of Neurosurgery. 2020;**134**(2):351–356. DOI: 10.3171/2019.11.JNS192224

[72] Neumann WJ, Gilron R, Little S, Tinkhauser G. Adaptive deep brain stimulation: From Experimental Evidence Toward Practical Implementation. Movement Disorders. 2023;**38**(6):937–948. DOI: 10.1002/mds.29415